Colleges of Medicine, Dentistry & Pharmacy

Kansas City, Missouri

Names of 3400 Graduates, 1871-1905

Compiled by

James A. Tharp MA, MLIS

March 2013

Tharp, James Alan (1946-)
  Colleges of Medicine, Dentistry and Pharmacy, Kansas City, Missouri: Names of 3400 Graduates, 1871-1905
    229 p.   cm.
    Includes bibliographical references and index.

ISBN-13: 978-0615770819
ISBN-10: 0615770819

1. Missouri–Biography. 2. Medical Schools. 3. Jackson County (Mo.) Genealogy. I. James Alan Tharp (1946-). II. Title.

Published by:
The Orderly Pack Rat
Kansas City, Missouri
david.jackson@orderlypackrat.com
www.orderlypackrat.com

Table of Contents

Introduction

Late nineteenth-century Kansas City, Missouri, was an active regional educational center for medicine, dentistry, and pharmacy. Students from Missouri and surrounding states formed the majority, but most other parts of the United States and Canada were also represented. During that period a bewildering array of medical and dental colleges existed in Kansas City, some continuing for decades and others lasting only a few years. That situation was further complicated by institutional name changes and mergers and removals across the Missouri-Kansas state line.

Allopathic, homeopathic, eclectic, and osteopathic approaches or "schools" of medicine were represented among Kansas City's early local institutions. Eventually, though, homeopathic and eclectic medicine declined in popularity and osteopathic education became firmly centered elsewhere, leaving primarily allopathic medical education in Kansas City.

Kansas City's early schools of medicine, dentistry, and pharmacy held annual commencement exercises honoring their new graduates, usually in March, April, or May. Newspapers usually reported those events, their reports varying widely in details covered. Some reported only the commencement's date or place. Sometimes the names of graduates who had been awarded prizes also appeared. In other cases, names of all graduating students were printed—occasionally even with their places of origin. Unfortunately, a few of the earliest commencements were not reported at all, but the customary use of phrases like "third annual commencement" in later reports implies the occurrence of those earlier unreported events.

This study focuses on the years 1871 to 1905, beginning with the first known commencement of a Kansas City medical school and ending somewhat arbitrarily in 1905, when several local medical schools merged to form the School of Medicine of the University of Kansas and by which time the list of graduates had become cumbersome.

Newspapers from 1871 to 1905 were searched intensively for reports of relevant commencements. The results were then assembled into a school-by-school chronological listing of more than 3,400 graduates based solely on those reports. An additional comprehensive alphabetical index provides for each graduate his or her school and year of graduation. Names of known school officials also appear in the index.

Finally, city directories of Kansas City, Missouri, were also consulted for each school's location, dates, and officers' names. A very brief historical sketch based on those data is provided for each school.

Additional articles about these schools were also located. While they are not included in the following bibliographic listings, copies of these articles may be researched at the Jackson County (Mo.) Historical Society Archives, Collection of Graduates of Colleges of Medicine, Dentistry & Pharmacy, Kansas City, Missouri, 1871-1905.

Central College of Osteopathy
(1903-early 1940s)

Central College of Osteopathy was founded in 1903 and its first known graduating class was in 1905. This college graduated several female physicians. It appeared in directories of Kansas City, Missouri, up through the beginning of World War II.

Surname	Given Names	City	State	Remarks
1905				
Courtney	Owen J.	Auburn	NE	
Green	Inez M.	Kirksville	MO	
Hailey	J. F.	Summit	MS	
Harding	Sallie (Miss)	Kansas City	MO	
Kreigh	Lutie (Miss)	Belton	MO	
Lindberg	B. W. (MD)	Kansas City	MO	
McKenzie	Lillian M. (Miss)	San Francisco	CA	
Mosbarger	James I.	Lincoln	NE	
Seaton	George M.	Lathrop	MO	

Newspapers

12 June 1904, the college building, Annual Commencement
"Reception to Students: Central College of Osteopathy to Close a Very Successful Year," *Kansas City (Mo.) Daily Journal,* 12 June 1904, section1, page 5, column 2. **(no list of graduates)**

22 June 1905, Central High School, Annual Commencement
"A Class of Nine Graduates: Central School of Osteopathy Held Commencement Last Night," *Kansas City (Mo.) Daily Journal,* 23 June 1905, page 10, column 2.
"Brief Bits of City News," *Kansas City (Mo.) Star,* 22 June 1905, page 10, column 1. **(no list of graduates)**
"Nine Osteopaths Graduated: Commencement Exercises of the Kansas City School Held Last Night," *Kansas City (Mo.) Times,* 23 June 1905, page 2, column 1.

21 June 1906, Central High School, Annual Commencement
"Osteopathy College Commencement," *Kansas City (Mo.) Star,* 16 june 1906, page 2, column 3.
    (no list of graduates)

27 May 1908, Spaulding's Hall, Annual Commencement
"Osteopathy to Be Graduated To-Night," *Kansas City (Mo.) Star,* 27 May 1908, page 3, column 3.

02 June 1910, Spalding's Commercial College, Annual Commencement
"Diplomas to Eleven Osteopaths," *Kansas City (Mo.) Star,* 13 May 1910, page 11, column 2.

30 May 1918, Grand Avenue [Methodist Episcopal] Temple, 16th [sic] Annual Commencement
"Graduates in Osteopathy: Exercises to Be at the Grand Avenue Temple May 30," *Kansas City (Mo.) Star,* 28 May 1918, page 12, column 4.

City Directories

1901 Kansas City, Missouri, directory   —
1902 Kansas City, Missouri, directory   —
1903 Kansas City, Missouri, directory, page 1497:
   [Full page display ad] Central College of Osteopathy, 729 Troost Avenue, Kansas City, Missouri. [Lists Board of Trustees, Officers of Board, Faculty for 1903-4, etc.]
1904 Kansas City, Missouri, directory, page 266:
   CENTRAL COLLEGE OF OSTEOPATHY 729 Troost office 432 New Ridge bldg Dr A L McKenzie pres Dr P M Agee v-pres Dr J N Parker dean [Also full page display ad page 1541]
1905 Kansas City, Missouri, directory, page 203:
   CENTRAL COLLEGE OF OSTEOPATHY 729 Troost tel Home Main 5305 office 432 New Ridge bldg Dr A L McKenzie pres Dr P M Agee v-pres Dr Geo Moffett sec Dr J W Parker dean [Also display ad, page 465]

College of Homeopathic Medicine and Surgery of the Kansas City University (ca. 1895-1900)

College of Homeopathic Medicine and Surgery of the Kansas City University was founded ca. 1895 and its first graduating class was in 1896. This college graduated several female physicians. In 1900 the school's name was changed to Hahnemann Medical College of the Kansas City University (1900-1902).

Surname	Given Names	City	State	Remarks
1899				
Bradley	Virginia A. (Miss)			
Coburn	Clay E.			
Doane	Florence E. (Miss)			
Northrup	John F.			
1900				
Bird	Arthur A.			
Bremen	M. Napier			
Church	Miriam Lyon (Mrs.)			
Irwin	George Elgile/Elgio			
Melton	Edgar A.			
Metzner	Alice P. (Miss)			
Mitchell	J. Frank			

Newspapers

21 March 1899, Lyceum Theater, 1st Known Annual Commencement
"Constantine Hering: Homoeopaths Honor One of Their Greatest Teachers—Address by Dr. Runnels," *Kansas City (Mo.) Daily Journal,* 18 March 1899, page 5, column 2.
"Kansas City Homeopathic College," *Kansas City (Mo.) Daily Journal,* 16 March 1899, page 7, column 3.
"Another College Commencement," *Kansas City (Mo.) Daily Journal,* 21 March 1899, page 3, column 4. **(no list of graduates)**

27 March 1900, Lyceum Hall, 2nd Known Annual Commencement
"More Commencements: College of Homeopathic Medicine and Surgery and Kansas City College of Pharmacy," *Kansas City (Mo.) Daily Journal,* 13 March 1900, page 7, column 4.
"Graduates in Homeopathy: Disciples of Hahnemann Receive Their Diplomas and Enjoy Good Music," *Kansas City (Mo.) Daily Journal,* 28 March 1900, page 3, column 3.
"Seven Doctors Graduated," *Kansas City (Mo.) Times,* 28 March 1900, page 6, column 3.

City Directories

1895 Kansas City, Missouri, directory   —
1896 Kansas City, Missouri, directory   —
1897 Kansas City, Missouri, directory   —
1898 Kansas City, Missouri, directory, Page 177:
    College of Homoeopathic Medicine and Surgery of the K. C. University, 903 Troost, Dr W H Jenney dean; Dr Frank Elliott sec; Page 967: College of Homoeopathic Medicine & Surgery of the K. C. University, 908 Troost. Dr. W. H. Jenney, Dean; Dr. Frank Elliott, Sec.
1899 Kansas City, Missouri, directory, Page 195:
    College of Homoeopathic Medicine and Surgery of the Kansas City University, 903 Troost, Gardiner Lathrop pres; Bruno Hobbs v-pres; W A Forster sec; Watt Webb treas; Page 1084: College of Homoeopathic Medicine & Surgery of the K. C. University, 908 Troost. Gardiner Lathrop, Pres; Bruno Hobbs, V-Pres; W. A. Forster, Sec; Watt Webb, Treas
1900 Kansas City, Missouri, directory, Page 226:
    College of Homoeopathic Medicine & Surgery of the K C University 903 Troost Dr W H Jenney dean Dr Frank Elliott sec; Page 1293: College of Homoeopathic Medicine & Surgery of the K. C. University, 903 Troost; Dr. W. H. Jenney, dean; Dr. Frank Elliott, Sec.

College of Physicians and Surgeons
(1870-1880)

College of Physicians and Surgeons was established in 1870 as a merger of Kansas City College of Physicians and Surgeons (1869-1870) and Kansas City Medical College (1869-1870). Its first graduating class was in 1870. In 1880 the school's name was changed to Kansas City Medical College (1880-1905).

Surname	Given Names	City	State	Remarks
1871				
Bowker	S. D.	Rosedale / Shawneetown		
Burdick	E. L.			
Connell	R. W.			
Conry	T. J.			
Gabriel	G. W.			
Holman	H. R.			
Smith	R. F.			
Tappan	F. A.			
Watson	John C.			
1872				
Dimmitt	J. P.			Ad Eundem Degree
Ellis	W. T.			
Keating	W. F.			
Robinson	W. H.			
Taylor	H. H.			
1873				
Goforth	E. G.	Westport	MO	
Miller	J. G.	Atchison	KS	Ad Eundem Degree
Sharp	Joseph	Kansas City	MO	
Swaney	Loren	Kansas City	MO	
Warring	J. W.	Stranger	KS	
Wood	Robert L.	Kansas City	MO	
1875				
Beard	J. M. G.	Oakwood	KS	Prize ($25)
Christy	A. C.	Sedalia	MO	
Grosshart	Joel E.	Bates County	MO	
Holt	A. T.	Waldron (Platte County)	MO	Prize ($100)
Hopkins	James A.	Stranger	KS	
Kesseler	A. T.		NY	
Morris	Wm. C.	Kansas City	MO	
Morton	D. K.	Kansas City	MO	

Surname	Given Names	City	State	Remarks
1876				
Bills	W. W.	Pleasant Hill	MO	
Gilliland	H. D.	Fredonia	KS	
Hernden	C. F.	Camden Point	MO	
Houston	F. A.	Pleasant Hill	MO	
Kennie	J. E.	Leavenworth	KS	
Limerick	S. B.	Kansas City	MO	
Osborn	William H.	Garnett	KS	Prize ($100)
Phillips	E. D. F.	Tonganoxie	KS	
Roberds	S. L.	Kansas City	MO	
Sheley	O. C.	Independence	MO	
Tyree	W. C.	Kansas City	MO	Prize ($25)
Van Hoy	J. H.	Index (Cass County)	MO	
Van Hoy	W. W.	Greenwood	MO	
Whipple	G. W.	Exeter	NE	
1877				
Bennett	R. S.	Pleasant Hill	MO	Valedictorian
Crinnian	J. A.	Kansas City	MO	Prize ($100)
Divelbiss	S. B.	West Point	MO	
Meek	Edward	Kansas City	MO	
Reece	W. D.	Hainesville	MO	
Schellack	A.	Fort Scott	KS	Prize ($25)
Williams	S. K.	Bates County	MO	
Woodson	Edward C.	Kansas City	MO	
1878				
Bond	M. M.			
Bragelton	J. B.			
Charles	A. Lester	Kansas City	MO	Prize ($100)
Coffey	J. L.			
Gilmore	E. G.			Prize ($25)
Gordon	H. S.			
Hayes	J. E.			
Smith	Ira W.			Prize (Books)
Washington	C. A.			

Surname	Given Names	City	State	Remarks
1879				
Gray	George M.	Kansas City	MO	
Hamilton	W. C.	Crab Orchard	MO	
Koons	Robert P.	Lazette	KS	
Lester	Charles H.	Kansas City	MO	
Lusher	Louis W.	Aubry	KS	
Mainhard	Eugene	Kansas City	MO	
Moore	F. M.	Perry	MO	
Rupp	David F.	Peoria	IL	
Smith	Ira	Butler	MO	
1880				
Adkins	James M.	Liberty	MO	
Allen	Eben N.	Rich Hill (Bates County)	MO	
Ashley	Walter H.	Lawrence	KS	Prize (Book)
Beeson	Henry O.	Spring Hill	KS	Prize ($100)
Cline	Isaac	Howard City	KS	
Cline	William B.	Howard City	KS	
Day	Sandusky A.	Osawatomie	KS	Prize ($25)
Goldsberry	Thomas M.	Wellington	KS	
Hulett	William H.	New Home (Bates County)	MO	
Kester	Josiah H.	Harrisonville	MO	
Minney	John E.	Kansas City	MO	
Morrison	Norman H.	Emporia	KS	Prize (Book)
Nichols	Fred G.	Howard	NE	
Northrup	Daniel B.	Valley Falls	KS	
Reed	Thomas A.	Kansas City	KS	
Schenck	Walter	Westport	MO	
Smith	George B.	Monterey	IL	

Newspapers

[unknown date] 1870, [unknown venue], 1st Annual Commencement

07 March 1871, Vaughan's Diamond Building, 2nd Annual Commencement
"Commencement Exercises of the College of Physicians and Surgeons," *Kansas City (Mo.) Daily Journal of Commerce,* 08 March 1871, page 4, column 4.

04 March 1872, Frank's Hall, 3rd Annual Commencement
"Commencement Exercises of the College of Physicians and Surgeons," *Kansas City (Mo.) Daily Times,* 05 March 1872, page 4, column 1.

14 March 1873, Frank's Hall, 4th Annual Commencement
"Medical College: Degrees Conferred Last Night—A Handsome Present," *Kansas City (Mo.) Daily Journal of Commerce,* 15 March 1873, page 4, column 4.
"Annual Commencement: Exercises of the Fourth Annual Commencement of the Kansas City College of Physician [sic] and Surgeons," *Kansas City (Mo.) Times,* 15 March 1873, page 4, column 1.

[unknown date] 1874, [unknown venue], 5th Annual Commencement

02 March 1875, Long's Hall, 6th Annual Commencement
 "Alma Mater: Kansas City Medical Institute, Dr. Schauffler's Address," *Kansas City (Mo.) Daily Journal of Commerce,* 03 March 1875, page 4, columns 2-5. **(no list of graduates)**
"Doctor's [sic] Doings: Annual Commencement Exercises of the Medical College," *Kansas City (Mo.) Times,* 03 March 1875, page 4, column 3.

09 March 1876, Frank's Hall, 7th Annual Commencement
"College of Physicians and Surgeons: Seventh Annual Commencement—Addresses Conferring Degrees," *Kansas City (Mo.) Daily Journal of Commerce,* 10 March 1876, page 4, columns 3-5.
"Commencement Exercises," *Kansas City (Mo.) Mail,* 10 March 1876, page 4, column 3.
"Commencement: A Large Audience Present at Frank's Hall Last Night," *Kansas City (Mo.) Times,* 10 March 1876, page 4, column 4.

06 March 1877, Frank's Hall, 8th Annual Commencement
"The Doctors: Eight New Ones Turned Out Last Night," *Kansas City (Mo.) Daily Journal of Commerce,* 07 March 1877, pages 4-5, columns 4-5, 1.
"Esculapian Exercises: Commencement Exercises of the Kansas City College of Physicians and Surgeons," *Kansas City (Mo.) Times,* 07 March 1877, page 4, column 5.

04 March 1878, Frank's Hall, 9th Annual Commencement
"Ninth Annual Commencement: Kansas City College of Physicians and Surgeons," *Kansas City (Mo.) Daily Journal of Commerce,* 05 March 1878, page 3, column 2.
"Nine New Doctors: At the Ninth Annual Commencement," *Kansas City (Mo.) Mail,* 05 March 1878, page 4, column 3.
"Medical Institute: Ninth Annual Commencement of the Kansas City Medical College," *Kansas City (Mo.) Times,* 05 March 1878, page 4, column 4. **(no list of graduates)**

04 March 1879, Second Presbyterian Church, 8th and 9th Streets), 10th Annual Commencement
"New Doctors: Commencement Exercises of the Kansas City College of Physicians and Surgeons Last Night," *Kansas City (Mo.) Daily Journal,* 05 March 1879.

"Doctor's Degrees: Tenth Annual Commencement of the Kansas City College of Physicians," *Kansas City (Mo.) Mail,* 05 March 1879, page 4, column 5.

02 March 1880, First Baptist Church, 11th Annual Commencement
"Seventeen Doctors: That Many Brand New Ones Were Turned Out Last Night," *Kansas City (Mo.) Daily Journal,* 03 March 1880, page 8, column 3.
"Physicians and Surgeons: [Sevent]een of Them Receive Their Sheepskins Last Night from Kansas City College," *Kansas City (Mo.) Times,* 03 March 1880, page 5, columns 1-2.

City Directories
1867 Kansas City, Missouri, directory   —
1870 Kansas City, Missouri, directory   —
1871 Kansas City, Missouri, directory, page 46:
     College of Physicians and Surgeons. J. K. Thacher, President; J. F. McAdow, Treasurer; E. W. Schauffler, M. D., Secretary; Vaughan's Diamond Building.
1872 Kansas City, Missouri, directory, page 52:
     College of Physicians and Surgeons. L. K. Thacher, President; J. F. McAdow, Treasurer; E. W. Schauffler, M. D., Secretary; S. S. Todd, M. D., President of the Faculty. Vaughan's Diamond Building.

1873 Kansas City, Missouri, directory, age 49:
    College of Physicians and Surgeons. L. K. Thacher, President; J. F. McAdow, Treasurer; E. W. Schauffler, M. D., Secretary; S. S. Todd, M. D., President of the Faculty; J. L. Teed, M. D., Secretary of the Faculty. Vaughan's Diamond Building.

1874 Kansas City, Missouri, directory, page 49:
    College of Physicians and Surgeons. L. K. Thacher, President; J. F. McAdow, Treasurer; E. W. Schauffler, M. D., Secretary; S. S. Todd, M. D., President of the Faculty; J. L. Teed, M. D., Secretary of the Faculty. Vaughan's Diamond Building.

1875 Kansas City, Missouri, directory, page 50
    College of Physicians and Surgeons. L. K. Thacher, President; J. F. McAdow, Treasurer; E. W. Schauffler, M. D., Secretary; S. S. Todd, M. D., President of the Faculty; J. L. Teed, M. D., Secretary of the Faculty. Vaughan's Diamond Building.

1876 Kansas City, Missouri, directory, pages 44-45:
    College of Physicians and Surgeons. L. K. Thacher, President; E. W. Schauffler, M. D., Secretary; S. S. Todd, M. D., President of the Faculty; EE. W. Schauffler, M. D., Secretary of the Faculty; T. J. Eaton, Treasurer of the Faculty. Diamond Building.

1877 Kansas City, Missouri, directory, page 45:
    College of Physicians and Surgeons. L. K. Thacher, President; E. W. Schauffler, M. D., Secretary; T. B. Lester, M. D., President of the Faculty; E. W. Schauffler, M. D., Secretary of the Faculty; T. J. Eaton, Treasurer of the Faculty. College Building, Main, junction Delaware.

1878 Kansas City, Missouri, directory, page 44:
    College of Physicians and Surgeons. L. K. Thacher, President; E. W. Schauffler, M. D., Secretary; T. B. Lester, M. D., President of the Faculty; E. W. Schauffler, M. D., Secretary of the Faculty; T. J. Eaton, Treasurer of the Faculty. College Building, Main, junction Delaware.

1879 Kansas City, Missouri, directory, page 47:
    College of Physicians and Surgeons. L. K. Thacher, President; E. W. Schauffler, M. D., Secretary; S. S. Todd, M. D., Dean of the Faculty; D. R. Porter, M. D., Treasurer of the Faculty. College Building, Main, junction Delaware.

1880 Kansas City, Missouri, directory, page 47:
    College of Physicians and Surgeons. L. K. Thacher, President; E. W. Schauffler, M. D., Secretary; S. S. Todd, M. D., Dean of the Faculty; D. R. Porter, M. D., Treasurer of the Faculty. College Building, Main, junction Delaware.

College of Physicians and Surgeons
of the Kansas City [KS] University (1894-1905)

College of Physicians and Surgeons of the Kansas City [KS] University was founded in 1894 and its first graduating class was in 1895. This college graduated several female physicians. In 1905 it merged with Kansas City Medical College (1880-1905) and Medico-Chirurgical College (1898-1905), forming School of Medicine of the University of Kansas (1905-).

Surname	Given Names	City	State	Remarks
1899				
Blewitt	W. F.			
Gannon	A. J.			
Greenlee	E. W.			
Hassig	J. F.			
Hogarty	Sadie H. (Miss)			
Scarlet	A. W.			
Scott	Anna J. (Miss)			
Sours	F. O.			
Tracy	Frank M.			
Walker	E. N.			
Ward	J. O.			
1900				
Anderson	C. L.			
Hartman	Milo E.			
Haynes	Elmer E.			
Kellam	S. H.			
Kuchard	D.			
Laslett	Elizabeth			
May	James W., Jr.			
McClintock	George			
McLaughlin	Chilton W.			
Mielke	Charles H.			
Moore	James M.			
Newlon	Will P.			
Northrup	Frank A.			
Omer	William J.			
Pattison	John F.			
Pfeffer/Pfeiffer	Silvia A. Luttrell			
Randles	Herbert			
Smith	D. E.			
St. John	Hugh R.			
Ultz	W. R.			
Wakeman	Frank J.			

College of Physicians and Surgeons of the Kansas City [KS] University
(continued)

Surname	Given Names	City	State	Remarks
1903				
Brainard	B. F.			
Clarkson	J. T.			
Conner	J. A.			
Fulton	J. A.			
Gerish	A. E.			
Orr	B. F.			
Powell	B. S.			
Stecher	H. E.			
Updegraff	C. D.			
Welch	James			
1904				
Barnes	Calvin			
Crooks	Charles H.			
Ensign	Charles F.			
Fahring	George H.			
Hall	L. R.			
Jones	J. Arthur			
Morrison	Robert L.			
Myers	J. L.			
Owen	S. Sheridan			
Stephens	T. C.			
Vermillion	J. N. S.			

Newspapers

[unknown date] 1895, [unknown venue], 1st Annual Commencement

[unknown date] 1896, [unknown venue], 2nd Annual Commencement

[unknown date] 1897, [unknown venue], 3rd Annual Commencement

[unknown date] 1898, [unknown venue], 4th Annual Commencement

28 March 1899, People's M. P. Church (KCK), 5th Annual Commencement
"They Finish with Honors: Eleven Medical Students Are Presented With Their Diplomas," *Kansas City (Mo.) Times,* 29 March 1899, apge 3, column 2.

27 March 1900, High School (KCK), 6th Annual Commencement
"Doctors Ad Libitum: Many Commencements Arranged for This Week—Programmes Arranged," *Kansas City (Mo.) Daily Journal,* 26 March 1900, Page 10, column 3.
"Twenty-One New Doctors: The Sixth Annual Commencement of the College of Physicians and Surgeons," *Kansas City (Mo.) Star,* 24 March 1900, page 9, column 3.
"New Doctors Get Diplomas: Twenty-One Young Physicians Complete Their College Course," *Kansas City (Mo.) Times,* 28 March 1900, page 3, column 4.

College of Physicians and Surgeons of the Kansas City [KS] University (continued)

[unknown date] 1901, [unknown venue], 7th Annual Commencement

[unknown date] 1902, [unknown venue], 8th Annual Commencement

25 March 1903, High School (KCK), 9th Annual Commencement
"Commencement Exercises: Ten Graduated from College of Physicians and Surgeons," *Kansas City (Mo.) Daily Journal,* 26 March 1903, page 5, column 4. **(no list of graduates)**
"Ten New Kansas Doctors: Commencement Exercises of the College of Physicians and Surgeons To-Night," *Kansas City (Mo.) Times,* 25 March 1903, page 5, column 1.
"Diplomas for Ten Doctors: Commencement Exercises of the College of Physicians and Surgeons," *Kansas City (Mo.) Times,* 26 March 1903, page 4, column 2. **(no list of graduates)**

31 March 1904, High School Auditorium (KCK), 10th Annual Commencement
"Doctors at a Banquet: The Festivities Preliminary to College of Physicians & Surgeons Commencement," *Kansas City (Mo.) Times,* 31 March 1904, page 4, column 3.
"Medical School Graduates: College of Physicians and Surgeons Holds Its Tenth Annual Commencement," *Kansas City (Mo.) Times,* 01 April 1904, page 1, column 2. **(no list of graduates)**

[unknown date] 1905, [unknown venue],11th Annual Commencement.

City Directories

1893 Kansas City, Kansas, directory   [not available]
1894 Kansas City, Kansas, directory   [not available]
1895 Kansas City, Kansas, directory   [not available]
1896 Kansas City, Kansas, directory   [not available]
1897 Kansas City, Kansas, directory   [not available]
1898 Kansas City, Kansas, directory   [not available]
1898 Young and Co.'s Business and Professional Directory, page 338:
    [Kansas City, Kansas] College of Physicians and Surgeons, Chamber of Commerce bldg.
1899 Kansas City, Kansas, directory   [not available]
1900 Kansas City, Kansas, directory   [not available]
1901 Kansas City, Kansas, directory   [not available]
1902 Kansas City, Kansas, directory, page 127:
    KANSAS CITY UNIVERSITY, Parallel w of Chelsea pl D S Stephens chancellor
1903 Kansas City, Kansas, directory, page 62:
    College of Physicians & Surgeons (Medical Dept K C University) Simpson junc Central, Dr J E Sawtell dean, H W Brown pres, Dr E M Hetherington sec, Dr Zachariah Nason, Dr R A Roberts treas
1904 Kansas City, Kansas, directory, page 66:
    College of Physicians & Surgeons (Medical Dept K C University) Simpson junc Central, W H Brown pres Peter Hughes v-pres C M Stemen 2d v-pres E M Hetherington sec R A Roberts fin sec Zachariah Nason treas J M Sawtell dean
1905 Kansas City, Kansas, directory, page 58:
    College of Physicians & Surgeons, Simpson junc Central, Dr P D Hughes pres Dr E M Hetherington sec Dr Z Nason treas.

Columbian Medical College
(ca. 1898-1901)

Columbian Medical College was founded ca. 1898 and its first graduating class was in 1899. In 1901 it merged into the Medico-Chirurgical College (1898-1905).

Surname	Given Names	City	State	Remarks
1899				
Bright	Henry F.			
Cook	Paul			
Farrow	Edgar A.			
Jackson	Bernard M.			
Smallwood	James J.			
Tout	L. D.			
1900				
Moore	William A.			
Palmer	Walter C.			
Rudbeck	John			
Wiley	Charles Zenas			
1901				
Bregoire	Joseph A.		MI	
Brookshire	William H.		MO	
Hughes	U. S. G.		KS	
Kelly	George Francis		MO	
Markin	Buyiman F.		IA	
Miller	John A.		Indian Territory	
Owen	Clay M.		KS	
Palmer	Thomas D.		OK Territory	
Patterson	William M.		KS	
Sims	Charles A. S.		MO	
Tout	Benjamin B.		MO	

Newspapers

27 March 1899, Lyceum Hall, 1st Annual Commencement
"Embryo Physicians," *Kansas City (Mo.) Daily Journal,* 25 March 1899, page 12, column 2.
"Six New Physicians: Receive Diplomas from Columbian Medical College," *Kansas City (Mo.) Daily Journal,* 28 March 1899, page 7, column 5.
"Its First Year Closed: The Columbian Medical College's Annual Commencement Exercises Last Night," *Kansas City (Mo.) Star,* 28 March 1899, page 12, column 1.
"These Men Will Cure Ills: Columbian Medical College Holds Its First Commencement," *Kansas City (Mo.) Times,* 28 March 1899, page 3, column 5.

19 March 1900, Academy of Music, 2nd Annual Commencement
"Columbian Medical College: Commencement Exercises and a Banquet to the Graduating Class Monday Night," *Kansas City (Mo.) Star,* 18 March 1900, page 4, column 1. **(no list of graduates)**
"They Are Doctors Now: Four Students Graduated from the Columbian Medical College," *Kansas City (Mo.) Times,* 20 March 1900, page 6, column 2.

19 March 1901, Academy of Music, 3rd Annual Commencement

"School Days Are Over: Commencement of Colombian [sic] Medical College at Academy of Music," *Kansas City (Mo.) Daily Journal,* 20 Marach 1901, page 3, column 2.

"Makes Eleven More Doctors: Diplomas Passed Around at the Columbian Medical College's Commencement," *Kansas City (Mo.) Star,* 20 March 1901, page 5, column 2. **(no list of graduates)**

City Directories

1897 Kansas City, Missouri, directory   —

1898 Kansas City, Missouri, directory   —

1899 Kansas City, Missouri, directory, page 1084:
    Columbian Medical College, 1729 Troost. S. G. Burnett Pres; G. W. Lilly, V-Pres; J. E. Morse, Treas; Geo. Morton, Sec; J. L. Robinson, Dean.

1900 Kansas City, Missouri, directory, page 1293:
    Columbian Medical College; 18th se cor Woodland; W. F. Morrow, Pres; P. C. Palmer, V-Pres; O. F. Jones, Sec; J. E. Moses, Treas; J. J. Robinson, Dean.

1901 Kansas City, Missouri, directory, page 234:
    Columbian Medical College 1801 e 18th

1902 Kansas City, Missouri, directory   —

1903 Kansas City, Missouri, directory   —

Dental Department of the Kansas City Medical College
(1881-1890)

Dental Department of the Kansas City Medical College was founded in 1881 and its first graduating class was in 1883. In 1890 it separated from the Kansas City Medical College and its name was changed to Kansas City Dental College (1890-1919).

Surname	Given Names	City	State	Remarks
1883				
Lane	David C.	Topeka	KS	
Root	Joseph P., Jr.	Wyandotte	KS	
1884				
Peck	J. W.	Olathe	KS	
1885				
Buchanan	James M.	Kansas City	MO	
Crozier	John E.	Lee's Summit	MO	
Dunning	William M.	Wyandotte	KS	Prize ($25)
Parr	Howard I.	Wyandotte	KS	Prize (Instruments)
Stark	J. K.	Kansas City	MO	Honorary Degree
1886				
Chipley	James N.			
Tullis	Morgan			
1887				
Earl	George W.			
Guss	James M.			
Heckler	John W.			
Lawrence	Robert			
McCarter	W. A.			
Nobles	Samuel S.			
Parsons	John H.			2 Prizes ($25 & Instruments)
Strickland	Frank			
1888				
Anderson	R. V.			
Leavel	J. L.			
Murdock	F. L.			Prize (Book)
Reavis	J. L.			2 Prizes ($25)
Reed	W. L.			
Smith	H. S.			Prize
Sweet	E. S.			
Tindall	C. M.			

Surname	Given Names	City	State	Remarks
1889				
Baum	Fritz			
Buchanan	Rice R.			Prize (Instruments)
Dickson	Benjamin H.			
Hannah	Jefferson D.			Prize (Instruments)
Hiatt	Newton W.			
Hughes	Horace J.			Prize (Book)
Larmer	Charles V.			
McKellar	Arthur E.			Prize (Book)
Thomas	Ross T.			
Warren	Frank L.			
Wheat	Samuel C.			Prize ($25)

Newspapers

06 March 1883, Walnut Street Methodist Episcopal Church (South), 1st Annual Commencement
"Commencement: Fourteenth Annual Graduation Exercises of the Kansas City Medical College—Addresses and
    Banquet," *Kansas City (Mo.) Daily Journal,* 07 March 1883, page 3, columns 1-3.
"Doctors Dine: The Commencement Exercises and Banquet Last Night," *Kansas City (Mo.) Star,* 07 March 1883,
    page 1, column 4.
"Medical College Commencement," *Kansas City (Mo.) Times,* 07 March 1883, page 8, columns 1-2.

04 March 1884, Coates Opera House, 2nd Annual Commencement
"'Healers,' Fifteenth Annual Commencement of the Kansas City Medical College," *Kansas City (Mo.) Daily
    Journal,* 05 March 1884, page 5, columns 1-5.
"Sixteen New Doctors: Fifteenth Annual Commencement of the Kansas City College of Medicine—The Exercises
    and the Banquet," *Kansas City (Mo.) Times,* 05 March 1884, page 8, column 1.

17 March 1885, First Baptist Church, 3rd Annual Commencement
"Medical and Dental Graduates," *Kansas City (Mo.) Daily Journal,* 18 March 1885, page 3, columns 2-3.
"Commencement Exercises," *Kansas City (Mo.) Star,* 18 March 1885, page 2, column 4. **(no list of graduates)**
"Fifteenth Commencement: Graduating Exercises of the Kansas City Medical and Dental Colleges—Prizes
    Conferred," *Kansas City (Mo.) Times,* 18 March 1885, page 8, column 3.

16 March 1886, Music Hall, 4th Annual Commencement
"More Doctors of Medicine," *Kansas City (Mo.) Daily Journal,* 17 March 1886, page 3, columns 1-2.
"Diplomas Awarded," *Kansas City (Mo.) Star,* 17 March 1886, page 1, column 7. **(no list of graduates)**
"Twelve New Doctors: Graduating Exercises of the Kansas City Medical College—Diplomas Awarded," *Kansas
    City (Mo.) Times,* 17 March 1886, page 8, column 2.
"Twelve New Doctors: Graduating Exercises of the Kansas City Medical College—Diplomas Awarded," *Kansas
    City (Mo.) Times,* 17 March 1886, page 8, column 2.

15 March 1887, Music Hall, 5th Annual Commencement
"College Commencement: Graduating Exercises of Two Kansas City Medical Institutions—Addresses Delivered,"
    Kansas City (Mo.) Daily Journal, 16 March 1887, page 4, columns 5-7.
"Twenty-Three New Doctors," *Kansas City (Mo.) Star,* 16 March 1887, page 1, column 1.
"Kansas City Medical Association," *Kansas City (Mo.) Times,* 16 March 1887, page 8, column 3.

13 March 1888, Music Hall, 6th Annual Commencement
"Commencement Exercises: Graduates in Medicine and Dentistry Receive Their Diplomas—An Address by Rev. Cameron Mann," *Kansas City (Mo.) Daily Journal,* 14 March 1888, page 3, columns 1-2.
"Doctors' Degrees: Graduation Exercises of the Kansas City Medical and Dental Colleges," *Kansas City (Mo.) Times,* 14 March 1888, page 8, column 3.

11 March 1889, Music Hall, 7th Annual Commencement
"Coming Events," *Kansas City (Mo.) Star,* 05 March 1889, page 1, column 4. **(no list of graduates)**
"The Twentieth Annual," *Kansas City (Mo.) Star,* 11 March 1889, page 2, column 7**(no list of graduates)**
"New Doctors and Dentists," *Kansas City (Mo.) Star,* 12 March 1889, page 1, column 2. **(no list of graduates)**
"Doctors and Dentists: Commencement Exercises of the Colleges of Medicine and Dental Surgery," *Kansas City (Mo.) Times,* 12 March 1889, page 2, column 3.

12 March 1890, Young Men's Christian Association Auditorium, 8th Annual Commencement
"Kansas City Dental College: Its Eighth Annual Commencement Held Last Night," *Kansas City (Mo.) Daily Journal,* 13 March 1890, page 2, column 3.
"Dental College Commencement," *Kansas City (Mo.) Star,* 12 March 1890, page 1, column 1. **(no list of graduates)**
"They Are Dentists Now: Sixteen Graduates from the Kansas City Dental College Receive Diplomas," *Kansas City (Mo.) Times,* 13 March 1890, page 3, column 2.

City Directories

1888 Kansas City, Missouri, directory   —
1889 Kansas City, Missouri, directory   —

Eclectic Medical University
(ca. 1898-1917)

Eclectic Medical University (Eclectic medicine) was founded ca. 1898 and its first graduating class was in 1899. This college graduated several female physicians. It last appeared in directories of Kansas City, Missouri, in 1917.

Surname	Given Names	City	State	Remarks
1901				
Bowen	C. W.		MO	
Briggs	I. Anderson		MO	
Gandy	Henry P.	Kansas City	MO	
Gilman	Charles J.	Kansas City	MO	
Hagenberger	Ida	Kansas City	MO	
Isley	Marques. D. S.	Excelsior Springs	MO	
Jaques	T. W.	Kansas City	MO	
Long/Lang	Minnie B.	Kansas City	MO	
McClelland	Charles A.	Kansas City	MO	
Reynolds	Elmer L.	Kansas City	MO	Valedictorian
Seymour	Darwin R.	Kansas City	MO	
Sherrer	May S.	Kansas City	MO	
Tucker	Harvey E.	Marshall	MO	
Williams	G. M.		TX	
Williams/Wilhelm	Levi R.	Kansas City	MO	
1903				
Barber	Arch L.			Salutatorian
Bean	George W.			
Castle	H. K.			
Francis	J. C.			
Howell	A. D.			
Martin	W. W.			Valedictorian
Meckfessel/Meckfessil	F. C./G.			
Myers	S. N.			
Patterson	B. J.			
Rinehart/Renehart	J. H.			
Sitton	William H.			
Tirchel/Trichel	J. J.			
Walsh	Thomas C./M.			
Yates	E. C.			

Surname	Given Names	City	State	Remarks

1904

Ball/Dail	James C.			
Billingsles	S. W.			
Dodson	John T.			
Drake	Lester M.			
Fellows	William R.			
Frazier	C. E.			
Gunston	Joseph R.			
Lowry	Joseph D.			
McCleary	A. S.			
Miller	Charles H.			
Page	Dolle			
Planck	Fred M.			
Reynolds	May			
Riggins	D. M.			
Williams	R. A. (MD)			
Young	W. H.			

Newspapers

[unknown date] 1899, [unknown venue], 1st Annual Commencement

[unknown date] 1900, [unknown venue], 2nd Annual Commencement

22 March 1901, Grand Avenue Methodist Episcopal Church, 3rd Annual Commencement
"Eclectic Medical: Third Annual Commencement Will Be Held Next Friday Night at Grand Avenue Church,"
    Kansas City (Mo.) Daily Journal, 20 March 1901, page 3, column 2.
"Eclectic's Commencement: Twelve Men and Three Women Graduated from the Medical University Last Night,"
    Kansas City (Mo.) Daily Journal, 23 March 1901, page 3, column 4.
"Another Grist of Medics: Kansas City Eclectic Medical University Graduated Fifteen New Doctors Last Night,"
    Kansas City (Mo.) Times, 23 March 1901, page 3, column 5.

[unknown date] 1902, [unknown venue], 4th Annual Commencement

13 March 1903, Academy of Music, 5th Annual Commencement
"Eclectic College Graduates: Twenty-Two Students Will Receive Their Medical Degree Tonight," *Kansas City
    (Mo.) Daily Journal,* 13 March 1903, page 5, column 7.
"Fourteen New Doctors: All Are Graduates of the Eclectic Medical University," *Kansas City (Mo.) Star,* 14 March
    1903, page 5, column 2.

24 March 1904, Academy of Music, 6th Annual Commencement
"Will Get Their Sheepskins: Class of Sixteen to Graduate from the Eclectic Medical University," *Kansas City (Mo.)
    Star,* 20 March 1904, page 2, column 2.
"Eclectic Medical College Commencement," *Kansas City (Mo.) Times,* 25 March 1904, page 2, column 4. **(no list
    of graduates)**

[unknown date] 1905, [unknown venue], 7th Annual Commencement

29 March 1906, Academy of Music, 8th Annual Commencement, "Brief Bits of City News," *Kansas City (Mo.) Star,* 28 March 1906, page 10, column 3.

City Directories

1901 Kansas City, Missouri, directory   —
1902 Kansas City, Missouri, directory   —
1903 Kansas City, Missouri, directory, page 371:
    Eclectic Medical University 1402 Grand av Dr Chas Palmer pres, Dr T L Noblitt v-pres, Dr S F March sec & treas
1904 Kansas City, Missouri, directory, page 363:
    Eclectic Medical University (1) 1400 Grand av Dr S F Marsh sec
1905 Kansas City, Missouri, directory, page 330:
    Eclectic Medical University (1) 1400 Grand av Dr F S March sec

Hahnemann Medical College of the Kansas City University (1900-1902)

Hahnemann Medical College of the Kansas City University (Homeopathic medicine) was formerly known as College of Homeopathic Medicine and Surgery of the Kansas City University (1896-1900). Its first graduating class was in 1901. This college graduated many female physicians. In the class of 1901, one (male) student from Japan was graduated. In 1902 this college merged with Kansas City Homeopathic Medical College (1888-1902), forming Kansas City Hahnemann Medical College (1903-1915).

Surname	Given Names	City	State	Remarks
1901				
Brooks	Lula Boling			
Brower	Asher A.			
Gibson	Bartlet Walter			
Kinley	Clarence Edward			
Mather	Joseph			
Maxson	Ira Lee			
McCoy	Charles Donald			
Smythe	Jay Bingham			
Wallick	Delbert LaZelle			
Wegman	William M.			
Yamada	Sigeru	Tokyo	Japan	
Youngman	Charles L.			
1902				
Bungardt	Carl Sperry			
Cowhick	Rebecca A.			
Dodson	John Francis			
Keeton	Rudolph Bascum			
Lindberg	Bernhard Waldemar			
Mehaffay	Andrew DeWitt			
Parker	John A.			
Simonds-Bash	Carolyn			
Wilhelm	Levi Robert			
Woods	Samuel Delos Evered			

Newspapers

26 March 1901, Lyceum Hall, 13th Annual Commencement

"Commencement Exercises: Hahnemann College Graduated Largest Class in Its History at Lyceum Hall Last Night," *Kansas City (Mo.) Daily Journal,* 27 March 1901, page 7, column 7.

"Diplomas for a Dozen Doctors: Twelve Were Graduated from the Hahnemann Medical College Last Night," *Kansas City (Mo.) Star,* 27 March 1901, page 9, column 1.

"Launched on Medical Sea: Twelve New Disciples of Hahnemann Given Diplomas at Lyceum Hall Last Night," *Kansas City (Mo.) Times,* 27 March 1901, page 6, column 4.

14 April 1902, Lyceum Hall, 14th Annual Commencement

"Homeopathic Graduates: Eight More Men and Two Women Are Now Entitled to Engage in the Practice of Medicine," *Kansas City (Mo.) Daily Journal,* 15 April 1902, page 5, column 3.

"Ten More Doctors to Graduate: Commencement Exercises of Hahnemann Medical College Monday Night," *Kansas City (Mo.) Star,* 13 April 1902, page 7, column 3.

"Ten More M. D's. [sic] Graduated: The Commencement Exercises of the Hahnemann Medical College," *Kansas City (Mo.) Times,* 15 April 1902, page 2, column 4.

City Directories

1901 Kansas City, Missouri, directory, page 446:

Hahnemann Medical College 561 Cherry Dr W H Jenney dean, Dr Frank Elliott sec

1902 Kansas City, Missouri, directory, page 481:

Hahnemann Medical College 561 Cherry, Dr W H Jenney dean

Kansas City College of Dental Surgery
(ca. 1885-?)

Kansas City College of Dental Surgery was founded ca. 1885 and its only known graduating class was in 1894. This school was accused of selling its diplomas to persons who had taken no classes. It last appeared in directories of Kansas City, Missouri, in 1897.

Surname	Given Names	City	State	Remarks
1894				
Atkinson	Cliff R.			
Blake	T. J.			
BrabawBraham	John V.			
Butterworth	J. M.			
Calhoun	W. S.			
Calmes	James B.			
Day	C. D.			
Groves	E. J.			
Keagle	Levi S.			
Mabee	O. P.			
Maberly/Moberly	E. H.			Valedictorian
Nicholson	George D.			
Randall	James J.			
Tibbals	E. R.			
Voorhies/Vorheis	R. C.			
Weaver	C. C.			

Newspapers

02 March 1894, Pythian Hall, 1013 Walnut Street, 1st Annual Commencement
"Sixteen Graduates: Commencement Exercises of the Kansas City College of Dental Surgery," *Kansas City (Mo.) Daily Journal,* 03 March 1894, page 8, column 3.
"Dental College News: The Annual Commencement Exercises of the Local Colleges," *Kansas City (Mo.) Star,* 03 March 1894, page 6, column 3. **(no list of graduates)**
"Sixteen Graduates: Commencement of the Kansas City College of Dental Surgery," *Kansas City (Mo.) Times,* 03 March 1894, page 2, column 5.

City Directories

1883 Kansas City, Missouri, directory   —
1884 Kansas City, Missouri, directory   —
1885 Kansas City, Missouri, directory, page 318:
    Kansas City College of Dental Surgery, 719 Main
1886-1888   —
1889 Kansas City, Missouri, directory
Page 369:
Kansas City College of Dental Surgery, J. T. Atkinson, dean 715 Main
Page 880:
    Kansas City College of Dental Surgery, J. T. Atkinson, Dean, 715 Main.
1890 Kansas City, Missouri, directory, page 937:
    Kansas City College of Dental Surgery, 500 Y. M. C. A. Bldg..

1891 Kansas City, Missouri, directory, page 863:
  Kansas City College of Dental Surgery 719 Main J. T. Atkinson dean
1892 Kansas City, Missouri, directory   —
1893 Kansas City, Missouri, directory, page 316:
  Kansas City College of Dental Surgery, 1017 Walnut J T Atkinson Dean
  Page 658:
  Kansas City College of Dental Surgery, 1017 Walnut
1894 Kansas City, Missouri, directory, Page 323:
  Kansas City College of Dental Surgery, 1017 Walnut, J T Atkinson dean
  Page 662:
  Kansas City College of Dental Surgery, 1017 Walnut
1896 Kansas City, Missouri, directory, page 383:
  Kansas City College of Dental Surgery, 4 e 10th J D Atkinson pres
1897 Kansas City, Missouri, directory, page 374:
  KANSAS CITY COLLEGE OF DENTAL SURGERY, 229 Nelson bldg. J T Atkinson sec
1898 Kansas City, Missouri, directory   —
1899 Kansas City, Missouri, directory   —

Kansas City [KS] College of Medicine and Surgery (1896-1898)

Kansas City [KS] College of Medicine and Surgery was founded in 1896. In 1898 it moved to Kansas City, Missouri, and changed its name to Medico-Chirurgical College (1898-1905).

Newspapers

26 March 1898, Midland Hotel, 1st Annual Commencement

"One Man Graduated: First Annual Commencement Exercises of the Medico-Chirurgical Medical College," *Kansas City (Mo.) Daily Journal,* 27 March 1898, page 3, column 5.

"Its First Year Closed: The Medico-Chirurgical College Holds Its Commencement Exercises," *Kansas City (Mo.) Star,* 27 March 1898, page 8, column 4. **(no list of graduates)**

"Confers Its First Degree: One New M. D. Is Turned Out," *Kansas City (Mo.) Times,* 27 March 1898, page 7, column 6.

City Directories

1896 Kansas City, Kansas, directory   [not available]

1897 Kansas City, Kansas, directory   [not available]

1898 Young and Co.'s Business and Professional Directory, page 338:

[Kansas City, Kansas] KANSAS CITY COLLEGE OF MEDICINE & SURGERY, (Dr Ernest P Lutz, dean; Dr James L Harrington, sec); Wyandotte bldg. Tel W 160

Kansas City College of Pharmacy
(ca. 1886-1898)

Kansas City College of Pharmacy was founded ca. 1886 and its first graduating class was in 1887. This college graduated some female pharmacists. In 1898 its name was changed to Kansas City College of Pharmacy and Natural Sciences (1899-early 1940s).

Surname	Given Names	City	State	Remarks
1891				
Brinkley	John A.	Kansas City	MO	
Chandler	John F.	Nebraska City	NE	
Holsinger	Susie (Miss)	Rosedale	KS	
Lowe	Otto W.	Kansas City	MO	
Maloney	Harvey J.	Shawnee	KS	
Maxson	John C.	Parsons	KS	
Miller	J. Harley	Kansas City	MO	
O'Keefe	Michael J.	Pierce City	MO	
Swope	Frank W.	Kansas City	MO	
Vanderpool	Edwin M.	Lathrop	MO	
Wickman	Erhard A./W.	Kansas City	MO	
1892				
Berry	Fred R.			
Bruning	Fred W.			Prize (Gold Medal)
Bryant	Frank			
Cannon	Robert			
Creach	J. C.			
Doyle	Fay E.			
Eyssell	William			
Gray	Corrie C.			
Hoover	J. B.			
Johnston	S. E.			
Lawson	C. W.			
Moses	Lottie (Miss)			
O'Brien	Frank			
Otterman	B. W.			
Paul	John B.			
Rybolt	J. B.			
Scott	S. E.			

Surname	Given Names	City	State	Remarks
1893				
Burns	Lee M.	Kansas City	MO	
Cox	Volney B.	Kansas City	MO	
Crampton	Fred L.	Kansas City	MO	
Cuddy	Joseph John	Riley	KS	
Entz	John C.	Hillsboro	KS	
Hecker	George J.	Montrose	MO	
Higgins	Arthur C.	Perry	IL	
Hinde	William B.	Oregon	MO	
Kridler/Kreidler	Alphonso T.	Kansas City	MO	
Kruger/Kreuger	Ralph L.	Kansas City	MO	
Morrison	Harry H.	Kansas City	MO	
O'Maley/O'Malley	James	Cincinnati	OH	
Richards/Richardson	William	Kansas City	MO	
Shirley	Edward E.	Augusta	KS	Prize (Gold Medal)
Shively/Shriveley	Albert L.	Stella	OH	
Wherritt	Hugh S.	Sheffield	MO	
Wolfe	John C.	Rich Hill	MO	
1895				
Arnold	Orion T.			
Cook	William O.			
Curry	Otto			
Frizell	L. N.			
Gilbert	Mary K.			
Gilbert	Richard O.			
Grindle	Mark R.			
Harris	Caleb B.			
Harrup	George B.			
Hirt	Emma			
Howard	Charles E.			Prize (Medal)
Jackson	Carl A.			
Janeway	James E.			
Jones	David G.			
Kinnard	James C.			
Miller	Charles J.			Prize (Medal)
Mitchell	Francis D.			
Posey	Harvey B.			Prize (Medal)
States	Hermann E.			
Stevens	R.			
Surface	Edgar M.			
Swearingen	William I.			
Welsh	Benjamin L.			
Weyant	H.			
Williamson	Sidney R.			
Wilson	Charles A.			Prize (Medal)

Surname	Given Names	City	State	Remarks
1896				
Baugh	Fred			
Branstetter	C. E.			
Broderick	F. C.			
Bunch	J. G.			
Chambers	James C.			
Chandler	John			
Clinton	Fred S.			
Cole	T. C.			
Comer	Dent R.			
Cunningham	Bell (Miss)			
Curtis	Nora B. (Miss)			
Hill	H. W.			
Hoernig	Ernest			Prize
Lyons	Robert J.			Prize
McNair	J. Sed			
Moore	G. S.			
Parker	O. T.			
Porter	F. L.			
Rawles	J. C.			
Reese	W. J.			
Roland	Harry E.			
Smith	George			
Smith	Thomas J.			
Tiernan	Theo G.			
1897				
Braun	Philip A.			
Chandler	John H.			
Chastain/Chastaine	Victor H.			
Cline	Frank			
Findlay	John A.			
Harris	H. I.			
Hassig	J. Frank			Valedictorian
Howell	Will Waddell			
Kepner	John Walter			
Mears	Edward W.			
Peabody	Ned J.			
Randles	Herbert			2 Prize (Gold Medals)
Richards	Howard H.			
Sanntrock	Toni (Miss)			Salutatorian
Shewmaker	James L.			
Swazy	J. Ernest			
Worthen	W. Jerome			

Surname	Given Names	City	State	Remarks
1898				
Armstrong	Eldon E.			
Barnes	Frank L.			
Benton	Harriet (Miss)	Odessa	MO	Prize (Gold Medal)
Crowder	William			
Donaldson	Clyde O.			
French	Fred W.			
Gates	Frank D./P.	Kansas City	MO	
Hall	James W.			
Johnson	John C.			
Klee	Theo. P.			
Lee	Richard E.			
O'Maley	George T.			
Preston	Walter E.			
Rawles	Alvin J.			
Reeves	Lester E.			

Newspapers

[unknown date] 1887, [unknown venue], 1st Annual Commencement

[unknown date] 1888, [unknown venue], 2nd Annual Commencement

[unknown date] 1889, [unknown venue], 3rd Annual Commencement

[unknown date] 1890, [unknown venue], 4th Annual Commencement

17 March 1891, Auditorium of the Young Men's Christian Association, 5th Annual Commencement
"Graduates in Pharmacy: The Fifth Commencement of the Kansas City College," *Kansas City (Mo.) Star,* 17 March 1891, page 2, column 7.
"Graduates in Pharmacy: Fifth Annual Commencement Exercises of the Kansas City College," *Kansas City (Mo.) Times,* 18 March 1891, page 4, column 6.

15 March 1892, Auditorium of the Young Men's Christian Association, 6th Annual Commencement
"Commencement Exercises: A Large Number Will Be Held during This Month," *Kansas City (Mo.) Daily Journal,* 09 March 1892, page 3, column 6. **(no list of graduates)**
"Graduates in Pharmacy," *Kansas City (Mo.) Star,* 16 March 1892, page 6, column 2. **(no list of graduates)**
"Graduates in Pharmacy: The Sixth Annual Commencement of the Kansas City College," *Kansas City (Mo.) Times,* 16 March 1892, page 8, column 3.

09 March 1893, Auditorium of the Young Men's Christian Association, [7th] Annual Commencement
"Seventeen New Pharmacists: Annual Commencement of the Kansas City College of Pharmacy," *Kansas City (Mo.) Star,* 09 March 1893, page 7, column 6.
"Given Their Diplomas: Graduation Exercises of the Kansas City College of Pharmacy," *Kansas City (Mo.) Star,* 10 March 1893, page 7, column 6. **(no list of graduates)**
"New Druggists: Graduating Exercises of the Kansas City College of Pharmacy—The Address," *Kansas City (Mo.) Times,* 10 March 1893, page 5, column 4.

[unknown date] 1894, [unknown venue], [8th] Annual Commencement

22 March 1895, Academy of Music, 9th Annual Commencement

"Graduates in Pharmacy: The College Commencement Programme Friday Includes a Speech by Mr. Tarsney," *Kansas City (Mo.) Star,* 21 March 1895, page 1, column 1.

"Graduates in Pharmacy: The Local College Gave Diplomas to a Class of Twenty-Six Last Night," *Kansas City (Mo.) Star,* 23 March 1895, page 8, column 2.

"Twenty-Six New Druggists: Ninth Annual Commencement of the College of Pharmacy," *Kansas City (Mo.) Times,* 23 March 1895, page 2, column 1.

10 April 1896, Academy of Music, 10th Annual Commencement

"Women May Make Pills: Two in a Class of Twenty-Four Graduated by the College of Pharmacy," *Kansas City (Mo.) Star,* 11 April 1896, page 8, column 2.

"Commencement Exercises: The Kansas City College of pharmacy Completes Its Tenth Year's Work," *Kansas City (Mo.) Times,* 11 April 1896, page 5, column 2.

15 April 1897, Academy of Music, [11th] Annual Commencement

"Seventeen Graduates: The College of Pharmacy to Hold Commencement Exercises Thursday," *Kansas City (Mo.) Star,* 11 April 1897, page 2, column 2.

"Pharmacists Graduated: Sixteen Men and One Young Woman Given Degrees," *Kansas City (Mo.) Star,* 16 April 1897, page 6, column 4. **(no list of graduates)**

"Handsomest Class of All: Kansas City College of Pharmacy Graduates Seventeen," *Kansas City (Mo.) Times,* 16 April 1897, page 6, column 5.

15 April 1898, Academy of Music, [12th] Annual Commencement

"Pharmacists to Be Graduated," *Kansas City (Mo.) Star,* 14 April 1898, page 9, column 5. **(no list of graduates)**

"A Woman Pharmacist: She Won Highest Honors at the Kansas City College of Pharmacy This Year," *Kansas City (Mo.) Star,* 16 April 1898, page 3, column 3.

"Druggists Get Degrees: Kansas City School of Pharmacy Graduates a Class of Fifteen," *Kansas City (Mo.) Times,* 16 April 1898, page 3, column 2.

City Directories

1885 Kansas City, Missouri, directory   —

1886 Kansas City, Missouri, directory   —

1887 Kansas City, Missouri, directory, page 821:
Kansas City College of Pharmacy, 12th, south-east corner McGee, Julius Schweitzer, president; S. Emory Lanphear, M. D., secretary.

1888 Kansas City, Missouri, directory, page 897:
Kansas City College of pharmacy, 911 and 913 east 10th. S. Emory Lanphear, president; R. R. Hunter, sec.

1889 Kansas City, Missouri, directory, page 880:
Kansas City College of pharmacy, 911 and 913 east 10th. S. Emory Lanphear, Pres.; R. R. Hunter, Sec.

1890 Kansas City, Missouri, directory, page 937:
Kansas City College of Pharmacy, 911 and 913 east 10th, S. Emory Lanphear, Pres. J. J. Keifer, Sec.

1891 Kansas City, Missouri, directory, page 354:
Kansas City College of Pharmacy, 913 e 10th

1892 Kansas City, Missouri, directory, page 326:
Kansas City College of Pharmacy, 913 e 10th

1893 Kansas City, Missouri, directory, page 316:
Kansas City College of Pharmacy, 913 e 10th J G Kiefer sec; W T Ford treas

1894 Kansas City, Missouri, directory, page 323:
Kansas City College of Pharmacy, 913 e 10th

1895 Kansas City, Missouri, directory, page 858:
Kansas City College of Pharmacy, 913 e 10th, D. D. Hamilton, pres.

1896 Kansas City, Missouri, directory, page 900:
Kansas City College of Pharmacy, 913 e 10th, A. Breunert, Pres.; R. R. Hunter, V-Pres; Julius Kiefer, Sec.; David Walker, Treas.

1897 Kansas City, Missouri, directory, page 887:

    Kansas City College of Pharmacy, 716 Delaware, A. Breunert, Pres.; R. R. Hunter, V-Pres; F. D. Mitchell, Sec.

1898 Kansas City, Missouri, directory, page 967:

    Kansas City College of Pharmacy, 714 Wyandotte. W. F. Kuhn, Pres; F. L. Crampton, V-Pres; F. D. Mitchell, Sec; David Walker, Treas.

Kansas City College of Pharmacy and Natural Sciences
(1899-early 1940s)

Kansas City College of Pharmacy and Natural Sciences was formerly known as Kansas City College of Pharmacy (ca. 1886-1898). Its first graduating class was in 1899. This college graduated some female pharmacists. Eventually this school dropped "and Natural Sciences" from its title; it appeared in directories of Kansas City, Missouri, up through the beginning of World War II.

Surname	Given Names	City	State	Remarks
1899				
Brown	John J.	Edmond	OK	
Ella/Ela	R. E.	Kansas City	KS	
Ermey	Charles W.	Fulton	KS	
Orr	Frank A.	Granger	TX	Prize (Gold Medal)
Robbins	Frank A.	White City	KS	
Rowell	Hiram J.	Excelsior Springs	MO	
Simonton	Thomas H.	Louisville	KS	
1900				
Avard	John Henry			
Bertholf	Charles M.			
Brown	Dennis J.			
Coughenour	John S.			
Irland	Robert Douglas			
Mugg	James Kelow			Prize (Gold Medal)
Wilkins	Calvin B.			
1901				
Cable	Kirk LeRoy		KS	
Carey	Clyde	Kansas City	MO	
Cartmell	Edwin Ruthbin		KS	
Cone	Norman Homer		KS	
Cyrene	John E.		KS	
Dorsey	Maurice Howard		KS	
Ellis	Lewis Orient		MO	
Hopper	Otto Blenn		MO	
Hunter	Nick		MO	
Jones	Charles Walter		MO	
Miller	Edward Payson		KS	
Peter	Fred Daniel		OK	
Pollock	Maude Alice		MO	
Reye	Edward George		NY	
Swaney	James		MO	
Tharp	Herbert Elmer		MO	

Surname	Given Names	City	State	Remarks
1902				
Bard	Shirley J.			
Barnhart	Earnest M.			
Casey	Fred G.			
Coan	Edwin E. N.			
Conrad	Joseph A.			
Davis	Harry R.			
Dockhorn	George H.			
Forcade	Lawrence H.			
Foulks	George W.			
Gardner	James W.			
Hay	Herbert H.			
Janney	W. J.			
Marsh	Alanson A.			
McNaught	J. Frank			
McNulty	Ralph W.			
Pettyjohn	Orpheus E.			
Shrauger	Oron J.			
Simpson	William N.			
Vincent	Earl D.			
Whitney	Minnie M. (Mrs.)			Prize (Gold Medal)
1903				
Barnhart	Elsie (Miss)			
DeLozier	J. M.			
Findley	Antoinette (Miss)			
Freisen	Jacob			
Gramley	Lee			
Kelly	Lottie (Miss)			
Lynch	Edward			
Parradowski	Joseph			
Poe	Guy			
Rennick	E. C.			
Roe	H. C.			
Roe	H. D.			
Sith	Roland R.			
Smith	Mame (Miss)			
Starnes	J. C.			
1904				
Cleeton	William F.			
DeGraw	Walter A.			
Dieter	Charles A.			
Drown	Earl E.			
Eyssell	Henry			
Fabian	Emil			
Ford	Marion B.			

Surname	Given Names	City	State	Remarks
1904 Continued				
Hamman	Thomas F.			
Hance	F. Alroy			
Hassig	Charles			
Hewitt	Charles R.			
Hudson	Carl H.			
Huyler	Frank M.			
Marak	Rudolph I.			
McGeorge	John I.			
Moore	Fred M.			
Myers	Samuel S.			
Parmenter	Earl L.			
Sloan	William B.			
Stoughton	Elgin L.			
Tancyhill	Thomas R.			
Taylor	Fletcher B.			
Williams	Herbert V.			
Wiswall	Cecil F.			
1905				
Harrah	Milo E.			
Prettyman	R. T.			2 Prizes (Gold Medals)
Also 16 Others				

Newspapers

13 April 1899, Academy of Music, [13th] Annual Commencement
"Seven New Pharmacists: The Graduating Exercises of the Kansas City College of Pharmacy Last Night," *Kansas City (Mo.) Star,* 14 April 1899, page 7, column 3.
"Drug Mixers Get Diplomas: College of Pharmacy and Natural Science Holds Its Commencement," *Kansas City (Mo.) Times,* 14 April 1899, page 5, column 3.

03 April 1900, Academy of Music, [14th] Annual Commencement
"Doctors Ad Libitum: Many Commencements Arranged for This Week—Programmes Arranged," *Kansas City (Mo.) Daily Journal,* 26 March 1900, Page 10, column 3.
 "College of Pharmacy Commencement," *Kansas City (Mo.) Star,* 02 April 1900, page 9, column 1.
"New Made Pharmacists: Seven Young Men Complete the Course at the Kansas City College," *Kansas City (Mo.) Times,* 04 April 1900, page 6, column 6.

27 March 1901, Academy of Music, [15th] Annual Commencement
"Sixteen New Pharmacists: Graduation Exercises of College of Pharmacy Took Place Last Night," *Kansas City (Mo.) Daily Journal,* 28 March 1901, page 3, columns 1-2.
"Nineteen More Doctors [sic]," *Kansas City (Mo.) Star,* 24 March 1901, page 5, column 2. **(no list of graduates)**

02 April 1902, Academy of Music, [16th] Annual Commencement
"Twenty New Dentists [sic]: Commencement Exercises of the Kansas City College of Pharmacy Held Last Night," *Kansas City (Mo.) Daily Journal,* 03 April 1902, page 9, column 2.

"School of Pharmacy Commencement," *Kansas City (Mo.) Star,* 01 April 1902, page 5, column 5. **(no list of graduates)**

"20 Pharmacists Graduate: The Commencement Exercises of the Kansas City College of Pharmacy," *Kansas City (Mo.) Times,* 03 April 1902, page 4, column 3.

02 April 1903, Academy of Music, [17th] Annual Commencement
"Pharmacy Graduates Dance: Alumni Association Entertained the 1903 Class at the Coates," *Kansas City (Mo.) Times,* 02 April 1903, page 6, column 4.

"Diplomas for Pharmacists: A Class of Fourteen Graduated from the Kansas City College," *Kansas City (Mo.) Times,* 03 April 1903, page 6, column 6.

31 March 1904, Academy of Music, [18th] Annual Commencement
"Commencement Exercises To-Night," *Kansas City (Mo.) Star,* 31 March 1904, page 2, column 2. **(no list of graduates)**

"Graduated Many Druggists: Commencement Exercises of the Kansas City College of Pharmacy," *Kansas City (Mo.) Times,* 01 April 1904, page 1, column 2.

"Pharmacists to Hold Graduating Exercises," *Kansas City (Mo.) World,* 30 March 1904, page 8, column 1.

29 March 1905, Academy of Music, 21st Annual Commencement
"Graduate Tonight: College of Pharmacy Students Will Receive Diplomas," *Kansas City (Mo.) World,* 29 March 1905, page 1, column 3. **(no list of graduates)**

"Pharmacy College Graduates: Diplomas Given to a Class of Eighteen at the Academy of Music Last Night," *Kansas City (Mo.) Times,* 30 March 1905, Page 4, column 2. **(no list of graduates)**

21 [or 14?] March 1906, Academy of Music, 22nd Annual Commencement
"Brief Bits of City News," *Kansas City (Mo.) Star,* 14 March 1906, page 8, column 2. **(no list of graduates)**

17 April 1907, Academy of Music, 22nd Annual Commencement
"Will Be Pharmacists Then: Graduating Exercises of the College of Pharmacy Wednesday Night," *Kansas City (Mo.) Star,* 15 April 1907, page 4, column 3. **(no list of graduates)**

_____ 1908, _____

06 May 1909, Academy of Music, 24th Annual Commencement
"Here Are 33 New Druggists: Commencement Exercises of the Kansas City College of Pharmacy," *Kansas City (Mo.) Times,* 07 May 1909, page 7, column 2.

City Directories

1899 Kansas City, Missouri, directory, page 1084:
   Kansas City College of pharmacy, 714 Wyandotte. W. F. Kuhn Pres; J. M. Love, V-Pres; J. R. Moechel, Sec; T. J. Eaton, Treas.
1900 Kansas City, Missouri, directory, page 1293:
   Kansas City College of Pharmacy, 714 Wyandotte. W. F. Kuhn, Pres; J. R. Moechel, Sec.
1901 Kansas City, Missouri, directory, page 580:
   Kansas City College of Pharmacy and Natural Sciences 714 Wyandotte, W F Kuhn pres, J R Moechel sec
1902 Kansas City, Missouri, directory, page 626:
   Kansas City College of Pharmacy & Natural Sciences 714 Wyandotte, W F Kuhn pres, J M Love v-pres, D V Whitney sec, F L Crampton treas
1903 Kansas City, Missouri, directory, page 640:
   Kansas City College of Pharmacy & Natural Sciences 714 Wyandotte J M Love pres, J P Reymond v-pres, D V Whitney sec, F L Crampton treas

1904 Kansas City, Missouri, directory, page 648:
   Kansas City College of Pharmacy & Natural Sciences 714 Wyandotte J M Love pres, J P Reymond v-pres, D V Whitney sec, H L Crampton treas
1905 Kansas City, Missouri, directory, page 605:
   Kansas City College of Pharmacy & Natural Sciences 714 Wyandotte J M Love pres Dr J T Mitchell vpres D V Whitney sec F L Crampton treas

Kansas City College of Physicians and Surgeons
(1869-1870)

       Kansas City College of Physicians and Surgeons was founded in 1869. It merged in 1870 with Kansas City Medical College (1869-1870), forming College of Physicians and Surgeons (1870-1880).

Kansas City Dental College
(1890-1919)

Kansas City Dental College was established in 1890; it was formerly Dental Department of the Kansas City Medical College (1881-1890). Its first graduating class was in 1890. In 1919 it merged with Western Dental College (1890-1919), forming Kansas City-Western Dental College (1919-?)

Surname	Given Names	City	State	Remarks
1890				
Barker	William Samuel			
Buckley	Alonzo Marion			
Campbell	James Reed			
Ewing	Frank Lund			
Gant	Charles Henry			
Gant	Samuel Martin			
Hawthorne	James Edmund			
Hutcheson	Robert Charles			Valedictorian
Johnson	Clarence Edgar			
McDonald	William Sherman			
Millett	Shirley Sexton			Prize (25)
Overstreet	Frank Lorenzo			
Phister	Henry Johnson			Prize (Gold Medal)
Sihler	Carl Ernest			Prize ($50)
Spruill	Charles Respass			
Williams	William Wallace			
1891				
Aitken	William K.			
Ashby	Alba L.			
Austin	Wallar B.			
Baker	William P.			
Baxter	Henry E.			
Buchanan	Wiliam C. K.			
Claypool	Frank J.			
Corey	Frederic G.			
Crow	Alonzo T.			
Detrick	Archie M.			
Draper	Charles A.			
Fowler	Rezin T.			
Galloway	James			
Gibson	Elbert Q.			
Greenlee	Robert P.			
Hale	William B.			
Hines	Harry E.			
Hitchens	Aaron L.			

Surname	Given Names	City	State	Remarks
1891 Continues				
Hunsicker	Franklin G.			
Kenney	Frank C.			
Kenney	James T.			
Kice	John D. V.			
Kincaid	Samuel W.			
Kirby	Augustine H.			
Laws	Paul J.			
Lewis	George L.			
Lyon	Charles B.			
Mann	Alfred H.			
McLeland	James R.			
Meyers	William B.			
Ockerman	Simpson			
Ockerman	William H.			
Park	Arthur D.			
Reed	Chester B.			
Roberts	Harry E.			
Sage	Albert O.			
Toler	Matt F.			
Upton	Winslow P.			
West	William W.			
Whitmer	Henry A.			
Wibking	Oakley R.			
Wilson	Frank M.			
Woods	George H.			
1892				
Amerman	George Washington			
Bagby	Arthur Hoffman			
Barton	Jefferson Davis			
Barton	Robert Edgar			
Blake	Frank M.			
Bredouw	Ludwig Henning			
Bryson	David Kerr			
Butt	James Whitehill			
Buttner	Johann Christian			
Campbell	John Malcolm/Malcomb			
Carter	Frank Lenoir			
Chase	Eugene Aquilla			
Cobb	Fred Lewis			
Cronkite	Fred Pierce			
Cross	Gustavus Montgomery			
Day	Charles William			
Dills	Irwin Wilson			
Doyle	Harry Mitchell			
Engel	Harry Baile			
Farnham	Amasa Holton/Molton			

Surname	Given Names	City	State	Remarks
1892 Continues				
Goodwin	James Henry			
Grant	Schuyler Colfax			
Griner	Oliver Tennyson			
Havely	Alanson Tuttle			
Highnote	Walter Emmitt			
Hopfer	Martin Henry			
Jenkins	John Howell			
Kelly	Henry Wilfred			
Kydd	John George Alexander			
Lindas	Henry Eugene			
Lindsey	Arthur Lee			
Lovell	Mark Chester			
McKee	William Amos			
Mitchell	George Daniel			
Neff	James Daniel			
Nelson	Clifford Howell			
Noble	Ernest Prindel			
O'Bryon	James William			
Pendleton	Daniel Franklin			
Renz	Samuel Joseph			
Smith	Ole Anderson			
Smith	Woodson Thompson			
Tetrick	George Leon			
Thompson	Charles Willetts			
Turner	Harry Hurt			
Tutt	Arthur Monroe			
White	Ned Elmore			
Wilhite	Pitts Elmore			
Williams	Frank Lincoln			
Woodside	John Bratton			
1893				
Davis	Andrew William			
Dwight	W. Harry DeWitt			Prize
Holke	John H. (MD)			
Winn	Richard Jefferson			Prize & Medal
1894				
Allen	Charles Channing			Prizes
Allendorph	Eugene Wesley			
Brady	James Burns			Valedictorian, Prize ($50)
Duncan	Harry Evert			
Galliher	John Hockaday			
Kinnan	Henry A.			
McKee	Joseph Edgar			

Surname	Given Names	City	State	Remarks
1894 Continues				
Millen	Richard Andrew			
Miller	James Arthur			
Pile	Schuyler Wallace			
Rathbun	Charles Nelson			
Reily	George Thomas			
Rothrock	Ellsworth L.			
Stote	Archibald Benjamin			
Thompson	Abram			
Wilkes	Augustus Morton			
1895				
Adcock	George Alfred			
Balthrope	Harry Wellman			
Barber	John			
Blackwell	Walter Eugene			
Bogue	Julian Colfax			
Branstetter	Theron Ives			
Brosman	William Henry			
Burns	George Robert			
Bush	Ferdinand John Henry			
Conrad	Edward Leo			
Curry	Amos Leo			Valedictorian
Cussons	Henry Ward			
Davis	Leland Payne			
DeBerry	William Angus			Prize (Instruments)
DeHaven	John William Henry			Prize (Gold Medal)
Furrow	William Edward			
Geenen	George Jretta			
Glenn	Charles Irwin			
Gwin	Walter Ray			
Longstreth	Joseph Thomas			
Lutz	Joseph			
McDonald	Samuel Myron			
Metzler	Milton Bird			
Miller	Jesse			
Munday	Franklin Kelay			
Needham	Charles Clay			
Nevitt	James Alexander			Prize ($25)
Newell	Thomas Glenn			
Palmer	Charles Mahlon			
Preston	Abram Pierce			
Prevost	Harry Lytle			
Riley	Frederick Harsh			
Saul	Overton Mathews			
Smith	Charles Newton			
Streicher	Albert Roman			Prize ($50)
Thompson	Arch			

Surname	Given Names	City	State	Remarks
1895 Continues				
Vaughn	John Walter			
Watkins	Eric Cephas			
Wright	Walter Zina			
1896				
Allison	Ernest Williams			
Baker	Daniel Boone			
Blakey	Ernest Marvin			Prize (Gold Medal)
Breck	Louis Merrick			
Brock	George Griffith			
Brown	Clarence Elmer (BS)			
Brumbaugh	Philip Grant			
Burner	Edwin Lee			
Copeland	James Fritts			
Davidson	Marshall Piper			
Driscoll	William Frank			
Enloe	Henry Vampool			
Griffith	Joseph Kimberlin (MD)			
Hall	William David			
Harford	Daniel Paul			
Hauser	George Frederick			
Heady	Henry Clay			
Hiner	Ed Morrison			
Jackson	Charles Delavan			
Kendall	Walter Estol			
Kingsley	Frederic Clayton			Valedictorian; Prize ($50)
Lowrey	Robert Denton			
Lux	George Philip			
Major	Sidney Moss			
Maxfield	Harry Borden			
Moore	LeRoy Wilburn			
Moore	Scott Roscoe			
Morgan	Edwin Adonijah			Prize (Gold Medal)
Morrow	Edwin Arthur			
Morrow	James Albert			
Morton	Edward Clarence			Prize ($25)
Palmer	Vernon George			
Poplin	Robert Lee			
Pound	Frederick Franklin			
Pribil	Frank Joseph, Jr.			
Roberts	Ira Alphonzo			
Scott	Aretas R.			
Shaw	Robert Thomas			
Shoop	Charles Victor			
Smith	David Newell			

Surname	Given Names	City	State	Remarks
1896 Continues				
Stote	Frederick Charles			
Terwilliger	Jesse Worrick			
Toler	Earle Dean			
Treyer	Edmond Joseph			
Watkins	Charles Franklin			
Wikoff	Charles Harrison			
Young	William Campbell			
1897				
Andrews	Arnelle D.			
Backus	Claude			Prize ($50)
Chalfant	Charles W.			
Colman	Guy C.			
Crawford	Wesley R.			
Cutler	William E.			
Davis	Freeman			
Dawson	James P.			
Engle	Howard S.			
Fessenden	H. W.			
Fields	Roger C.			
Graham	James H.			
Gwinn	Mark D.			
Hart	Clinton T.			
Hopkins	Charles L.			
Hults	A. P.			
Johnson	Shelley K.			
Keith	James T.			
Kelly	Thaddeus S.			
Kittell	George H.			
Koger	Leonard D.			
Larmer	Curtis L.			
Leviston	F. E.			
McCarty	C. B.			
Moore	William A.			
Netherton	John W.			
Nipps	William H.			Prize ($25)
Numbers	Simon G.			
Pancoast	Clyde M.			
Pendleton	R. H.			
Purcell	Thomas E.			
Reily	John A.			
Rogers	Elby D.			
Ruddell	George, Jr.			
Seyster	George C./O.			
Smith	W. S. T.			Prize (Medal)
Stiles	E. H., Jr.			
Wilson	John T.			
Winkler	Elijah G.			

Surname	Given Names	City	State	Remarks
1898				
Ames	Adelbert David			
Baker	George Arthur			
Caldwell	Francis Marion			
Charlston	Oscar Oliver Solomon			
Cockrill	Thomas Monroe			Salutatorian
Dampf	John A.			
Dodds	William Evans			
Esterly	George Aden			
Foster	Benjamin Lombard			
Glasscock	Frank Ashton			
Hardy	James Edward			
Henderlider	Earl A.			
Kapitan	Emil Marvin			
Kerns	Andrew Franklin			
McCrary	William B.			
McDowell	Edward Theodore			
Miller	Ed A.			
Payfair	Tracy Morgan			
Ramsey	Thomas Bracken			
Schumann	Washington Egan			
Seibel	Richard Moritz			
Shackelford	Werter Davis			
Shewmaker	James Ezra			
Shrock	Earl Waldow			
Ward	George Walton			
Waters	Henry M.			
Wenker	Benedict George			
Wheeler	Edouardo Panschaud			
Wherry	Styles Winter			
Woods	Dixon Holliday			
Yager	John Calvin			
Yingling	Frederick Manassen			
1899				
Austin	Daniel Milton			
Bamber	John William			
Beaumont	Francis Hugh			
Bentz	Peter J.			
Bull	Clyde Westcott			
Caldwell	William L.			
Chenoweth	Robert Atkinson			
Cowdery	John Ray			
Davis	Loyd			
Haldeman	Oliver Cowdery			
Hargis	William Harrison			

Surname	Given Names	City	State	Remarks
1899 Continues				
Hocker	Clarence Eugene Elsworth			
House	Charles Henry Harry			
Hults	Milton Irwin			Prize (Instruments)
Hunger	Ferdinand Jacob			
Letord	Henri			3 Prizes (Gold Medal & Instruments)
Martin	Claude Anderson			Prize ($50)
Mathers	Edgar Randolph			
McAntire	Clarence Arthur			
McKee	Robert Stephenson			
Miller	Moses Alexander			
Pennock	Oscar Adrian			
Swisher	William Anthony			
Wells	Owen Delbert			Prize (Instruments)
1900				
Austin	William Earle			
Bishop	John K.			Prize ($50)
Bowers	Robert Harry			
Connolly	Charles L.			
Dillon	John A.			Prize (Instruments)
Enloe	Henry King			
Gants	Del Monte Timothy			
Gossard	Albert Edward			
Hazen	Calvin Edward			
Humfreville	George Bronson			
Iserman	Fred Eugene			
Keim	George Herbert			
Loring	Ernest Linwood			
Mayes	Claude LaFaun			
McCue	William Edward			
Michaels	Adolph Bancroft			
Park	Jerman Christy			
Pierce	Eugene Beecher			Prize (Instruments)
Robertson	Thomas Meade			
Stratton	Alfred Clinton			Prizes ($25, Gold Medal, etc.)
Tomiska	Joseph			
Walker	David			
Warner	Charles Pomeroy			
Weddle	Harold Christian			
Wertz	George Deal			

1901
33 Graduates

Surname	Given Names	City	State	Remarks
1903				
Allen	Frank Elwood			3 Prizes (Gold Medals)
Bamford/Mamford	Hubert M.			
Boehringer	G. J.			
Bonar	Earl Archibald			
Briggs	Charles R.			
Burnett	Clyde Bellamy			
Campbell	Edward O.			
Canoyer	Fenton M.			
Curtis	Joel A.			
Enloe	Enoch D.			
Enloe	Fred H.			
Feese	Edwin L.			
Grandstaff	Roy W.			
Hall	Edouard M.			
Hanna	Smith B.			
Kennedy	Ernest W.			
McCue	Virgil R.			
McFarland	Frank M.			
McKee	Harry H.			
Miller	Marvin B.			
Painton	Mark James			2 Prizes (Gold Medal)
Proffitt	James Hanson			Prize
Reed	John T.			
Robertson	John Q.			
Smith	Otis L.			
Tesch	Claude O.			
Waring	Andrew Bruce			Prize (Gold Medal)
Weston	Arthur F.			
1905				
Ballou	Emery H.			
Beeler	Charles E.			
Benton	Atwell L.			
Bussard	Bertram A.			
Coggins	John W.			
Collins	Thomas J.			
Combs	Frederick D.			
Dillman	Lawrence			
Drake	Joseph A.			
Dyer	Joseph H.			
Elder	Clifford D.			
Ellis	Claude			
Gahagen	Jay C.			
Gilley	Henry D.			
Graham	Percy Bruce			2 Prizes
Gregory	William Edward			Prize
Hanson	Swend A.			

Surname	Given Names	City	State	Remarks

1905 Continues

Surname	Given Names
Helm	John J.
Hunter	Durward B.
Hunter	Elmer A.
Johnson	Albert S.
Keys	William J.
Leonard	Alfred W.
Matthews	Roy M.
McBride	William H.
O'Bryon	Calvin F.
Osborn	Samuel E.
Petry	William B.
Pugh	William H.
Sager	Homer A.
Shally	George W.
Smith	Jay W.
Snyder	George B.
Sperry	Edward B.
Speyer	Maurice M.
Stewart	Samuel H.
Stone	Joshua R.
Swaney	Louis M.
Thimes	John W.
Watkins	A. Todd
Watson	Guy I.
West	Arthur J.
Wilcox	Frank B.
Wilkening	William A. N.
Williams	Daniel L.
Wilson	Clarence D.
Workman	Clarence B.
Zimmerman	John E.

Newspapers

10 March 1891, Grand Avenue Methodist Episcopal Church, 9th Annual Commencement
"News of the Medical Schools," *Kansas City (Mo.) Star,* 10 March 1891, page 3, column 3. **(no list of graduates)**
"Graduates in Dentistry," *Kansas City (Mo.) Star,* 11 March 1891, page 3, column 6. **(no list of graduates)**
"Graduates in Dentistry: Commencement Exercises of the Kansas City Dental College," *Kansas City (Mo.) Times,* 11 March 1891, page 8, column 4.

04 March 1892, Grand Avenue Methodist Episcopal Church, 10th Annual Commencement
"The Dental College: Its Tenth Annual Commencement Exercises Followed by a Banquet," *Kansas City (Mo.) Daily Journal,* 05 March 1892, page 8, column 3.
"Local Notices," *Kansas City (Mo.) Star,* 01 March 1892, page 4, column 7. **(no list of graduates)**
"Young Doctors: A Big Class Turned Out by the Kansas City Dental College," *Kansas City (Mo.) Times,* 05 March 1892, page 3, column 4.

03 March 1893, Coates House Hotel, 11th Annual Commencement
"Dentists Banquet: They Try Their Teeth on the Delicacies of the Season," *Kansas City (Mo.) Daily Journal,* 04 March 1893, page 3, column 1.
"Graduates in Dentistry: Banquet and Commencement of the Kansas City Dental College," *Kansas City (Mo.) Star,* 04 March 1893, page 8, column 1.
"Think of the Suffering! One Party Has Endured It, the Other Will Inflict It," *Kansas City (Mo.) Times,* 04 March 1893, page 2, column 1.

05 March 1894, Grand Avenue Methodist Episcopal Church, 12th Annual Commencement
"Prizes and Diplomas: Sixteen Graduates in Dental Surgery Listen to an Interesting Historical Sketch," *Kansas City (Mo.) Daily Journal,* 06 March 1894, page 8, column 2.
"Sixteen New Dentists," *Kansas City (Mo.) Star,* 06 March 1894, page 6, column 1.

01 March 1895, Auditorium Theater, 13th Annual Commencement
"Graduates in Dentistry: The Kansas City Dental College Holds Its Thirteenth Annual Commencement—The Banquet," *Kansas City (Mo.) Daily Journal,* 02 March 1895, page 3, column 2.
"Diplomas for Dental Students: Exercises of the Kansas City College at the Auditorium Last Night," *Kansas City (Mo.) Star,* 02 March 1895, page 2, column 1.
"Dental Grads: Annual Commencement and Banquet Held Last Night," *Kansas City (Mo.) Times,* 02 March 1895, page 5, column 4.

31 March 1896, Auditorium Theater, 14th Annual Commencement
"Dentists Turned Loose: A Class of Forty-Seven Graduated Last Evening," *Kansas City (Mo.) Daily Journal,* 01 April 1896, page 5, column 4.
"Forty-Seven New Dentist: The Eleventh Annual Commencement of the Kansas City Dental College Is Held," *Kansas City (Mo.) Star,* 01 April 1896, page 8, column 2.
"Knights of the Forceps: Forty-Seven New Dentists Graduated Last Night," *Kansas City (Mo.) Times,* 01 April 1896, page 7, columns 3-4.

31 March 1897, Coates Opera House, 15th Annual Commencement
"Dental Surgery Doctors: This Degree Conferred upon 39 Young Men Last Night," *Kansas City (Mo.) Daily Journal,* 01 April 1897, page 3, column 5.
"Thirty-Nine New Dentists: The Commencement Exercises of the Kansas City Dental College Last Night," *Kansas City (Mo.) Star,* 01 April 1897, page 8, column 2.
"Ready to Fill and Pull: Thirty-Nine Graduates Turned Out by the Kansas City Dental College," *Kansas City (Mo.) Times,* 01 April 1897, page 6, column 4. **(no list of graduates)**

05 April 1898, Coates Opera House, 16th Annual Commencement
"Dentists Given Degrees: Annual Commencement of Kansas City Dental College," *Kansas City (Mo.) Daily Journal,* 06 April 1898, page 5, column 6.
"More Young Dentists: Thirty-Two Tooth-Pullers Graduated by the Kansas City Dental College," *Kansas City (Mo.) Star,* 06 April 1898, page 4, column 7. **(no list of graduates)**
"May Fill Teeth Now: Large Class Is Graduated from Kansas City Dental College," *Kansas City (Mo.) Times,* 06 April 1898, page 6, column 2.

01 April 1899, Coates Opera House, 17th Annual Commencement
"Kansas City Dental College," *Kansas City (Mo.) Daily Journal,* 26 March 1899, page 3, column 2.
"Doctor of Dentistry: Degree Conferred upon Many Last Night," *Kansas City (Mo.) Daily Journal,* 02 April 1899, page 3, columns 4-5.
"Brief Bits of City News," *Kansas City (Mo.) Star,* 31 March 1899, page 2, column 5.
"Doctors of Dental Surgery: Kansas City Dental College Commencement," *Kansas City (Mo.) Times,* 02 April 1899, page 3, column 5.

30 April 1900, Academy of Music, 18th Annual Commencement
"Two Commencements: Two Colleges Have Closed Their School Year," *Kansas City (Mo.) Daily Journal,* 01 May 1900, page 9, column 5.

"Twenty-Six New Dentists," *Kansas City (Mo.) Star,* 30 April 1900, page 2, column 4.
"Many Dentists Turned Out: Kansas City College Graduates a Large Class," *Kansas City (Mo.) Times,* 01 May 1900, page 5, column 2.

29 April 1901, Coates House Hotel, 19th Annual Commencement
"Dentists' Annual Spread: Kansas City Dental College Holds Banquet at the Coates Hotel," *Kansas City (Mo.) Daily Journal,* 30 April 1901, page 1, column 2. **(no list of graduates)**
"Were Both Fed and Graduated: Diplomas Distributed at a Banquet to Thirty-Three Dental Students," *Kansas City (Mo.) Star,* 30 April 1901, page 10, column 2. **(no list of graduates)**
"Dentists at a Banquet: Faculty and Students Surrounded the Festive Board," *Kansas City (Mo.) Times,* 30 April 1901, page 3, column 6. **(no list of graduates)**

[unknown date] 1902, [unknown venue], 20th Annual Commencement

04 May 1903, Central High School, 20th [i.e. 21st] Annual Commencement
"Twenty-Eight New Dentists: Graduation Exercises of Kansas City Dental College Last Night," *Kansas City (Mo.) Daily Journal,* 05 May 1903, page 5, column 4.
"Twenty-Eight New Dentists: Annual Commencement Exercises of the Kansas City Dental College," *Kansas City (Mo.) Times,* 05 May 1903, page 6, column 3.

[unknown date] 1904, [unknown venue], 22nd Annual Commencement

11 May 1905, Central High School, 15th Annual Commencement
"Forty-Eight New Dentists: Commencement Exercises of the Kansas City College Last Night," *Kansas City (Mo.) Times,* 12 May 1905, page 5, column 2.

City Directories

1890 Kansas City, Missouri, directory, page 374:
    Kansas City Dental College, 500-505 Y. M. C. A. bldg
1891 Kansas City, Missouri, directory, page 354;
    Kansas City Dental College, 500-505 Y. M. C. A. bldg
1892 Kansas City, Missouri, directory, page 326:
    Kansas City Dental College, 500 Y M C A bldg
1893   —
1894 Kansas City, Missouri, directory, page 323:
    Kansas City Dental College, 10th nw cor Troost, C B Hewitt pres; J D Patterson sec
1895 Kansas City, Missouri, directory, page 365:
    Kansas City Dental College, 10th nw cor Troost, J D Patterson sec
1896 Kansas City, Missouri, directory, page 383:
    Kansas City Dental College, 930 Troost, J D Patterson sec
1897 Kansas City, Missouri, directory, page 374:
    KANSAS CITY DENTAL COLLEGE, 930 Troost, J D Patterson sec
1898 Kansas City, Missouri, directory, page 410:
    KANSAS CITY DENTAL COLLEGE, 930 Troost, A H Thompson, Topeka, Kas, pres; J D Patterson sec; W T Stark treas
1899 Kansas City, Missouri, directory, page 458:
    Kansas City Dental College, 930 Troost, S P Larmer Albany Mo pres; J D Patterson sec; W T Stark treas
1900 Kansas City, Missouri, directory, page 539:
    Kansas City Dental College 1024 e 10th S P Larmer pres, J M Austin first vice-pres, A Doud sec v-pres, J D Patterson sec, W T Stark treas
1901 Kansas City, Missouri, directory, page 580:
    Kansas City Dental College 1024 e 10th nw cor Troost Dr J M Austin pres, Dr J D Patterson sec, Dr W T Stark treas

1902 Kansas City, Missouri, directory, page 626:
Kansas City Dental College 1024 e 10th nw cor Troost, Dr J D Patterson pres, Dr W T Stark treas, C C Allen sec
1903 Kansas City, Missouri, directory, page 640:
Kansas City Dental College Troost sw cor 10th J D Patterson pres, W T Stark treas C C Allen sec
1904 Kansas City, Missouri, directory, page 648:
KANSAS CITY DENTAL COLLEGE Troost nw cor 10th J D Patterson pres W T Stark treas C C Allen sec
1905 Kansas City, Missouri, directory, page 605:
KANSAS CITY DENTAL COLLEGE 1024 e 10th sec office 510 Rialto bldg Dr J D Patterson pres Dr C C Allen sec Dr W T Stark treas

Kansas City Hahnemann Medical College
(1902-1915)

Kansas City Hahnemann Medical College (Homeopathic medicine) was established in 1902 as a merger of Kansas City Homeopathic Medical College (1888-1902) and Hahnemann Medical College of the Kansas City University (1900-1902). Its first graduating class was in 1903. This school last appeared in directories of Kansas City, Missouri, in 1915.

Surname	Given Names	City	State	Remarks
1903				
Brooks/Brooke	James Frank			
Cady	Frances A.			
Carter	Lew Arthur			
Coleman	William Orange			
Fuller	Silvies S.			
Gammage	Tom Rogers			
Luff	Joseph			
Miller	Enoch Merrill			
Puckett	Gladys Colt			
Reynolds	Oscar Hugh Wiley			
Richardson	Ira Frederick			
Riddle	Cordelia Alida			
Robinson	Samuel Sheldon			
Schoor	Albert Henry			
Welsh	Luther Winfield			
Williams	Reuben Augustine			
Young	Herbert Earl			

Newspapers

09 April 1903, Academy of Music, 15th Annual Commencement
"Another Class of Doctors: Commencement Exercises of Hahnemann Medical College," *Kansas City (Mo.) Times,* 07 April 1903, page 6, column 2.
"Homeopathic Graduates: Diplomas for Seventeen New Doctors Were Given Last Night," *Kansas City (Mo.) Times,* 10 April 1903, page 5, column 2.

08 April 1904, Academy of Music, 16th Annual Commencement
"Turning Out New Doctors: Sixteenth Annual Commencement of Hahnemann Medical College," *Kansas City (Mo.) Daily Journal,* 05 April 1904, page 5, column 5. **(no list of graduates)**
"Hahnemann Commencement Exercises," *Kansas City (Mo.) Star,* 06 April 1904, page 10, column 5.
"Homeopathic Physicians: Commencement Exercises Friday Night of the Hahneman [sic] College," *Kansas City (Mo.) Times,* 05 April 1904, page 7, column 4. **(no list of graduates)**
"Medical College Graduates: Hahnemann Medical School Issues Diplomas to Forty-Two [sic]," *Kansas City (Mo.) Times,* 09 April 1904, page 2, column 2. **(no list of graduates)**

[unknown date] 1905, [unknown venue], 17th Annual Commencement

"Hahnemann Commencement Exercises," *Kansas City (Mo.) Star,* 06 April 1906, page 10, column 5.

City Directories

1901 Kansas City, Missouri, directory   —
1902 Kansas City, Missouri, directory   —
1903 Kansas City, Missouri, directory, Page 641:
> Kansas City Hahnemann Medical College 1020 e 10th S H Anderson dean, M T Runnels registrar, Wm Craemer treas & bus mgr
> Page 499:
> Hahnemann Medical College 1020 e 10th S H Anderson pres, M T Runnels sec, W E Cramer treas

1904 Kansas City, Missouri, directory, page 499:
> Hahnemann Medical College 1020 e 10th Dr Chas Ott pres Dr Moses T Runnels dean Dr B B Andrews registrar Dr W E Cramer treas Dr D S Stephens chancellor

1905 Kansas City, Missouri, directory, page 606:
> Kansas City Hahnemann Medical College 1020 e 10th Dr Chas Ott pres Dr Frank Elliott dean Dr G W Smith registrar Dr E H Merwin treas Dr D S Stephens chancellor Dr J M Patterson v-pres Dr W A Forster sec

Kansas City Homeopathic Medical College
(1888-1902)

     Kansas City Homeopathic Medical College was founded in 1888 and its first graduating class was in 1889. This college graduated many female physicians. In 1902 it merged with Hahnemann Medical College of the Kansas City University (1900-1902), forming Kansas City Hahnemann Medical College (1903-1915).

Surname	Given Names	City	State	Remarks
1889				
Dassler	P. H.	Kansas City	MO	
Hall	B. F.	Phillips County	KS	
Stafford	A. M.	Independence	MO	
Vasbury	W. D.	Kansas City	MO	
1890				
Doane	Helen C. (Mrs.)			
Freeborn	Grant			
Green	Mary J. (Mrs.)			Valedictorian
Hickey	L. (Mrs.)			
Norris	E. L. (Mrs.)			
Van Meer	William			
1891				
Black	Charles D.	Argentine	KS	
Cookingham	Darwin A.	McPherson	KS	
Dewar	Hugh M.	London	ON	
Horton	Warner H.	Belmont	IA	
Ray	William L.	Pleasant Hill	MO	
Schoor	Edward/Edwin	Garden City	MO	
1892				
Cline	P. (Miss)	Kansas City	MO	
DeWolf	F. L.	Girard	KS	
Peet	P. F.	New York	NY	
Radley	James K.	Kansas City	MO	
Seeger	E.	Kansas City	MO	
1893				
Ball	James			
Billings	Robert A.			
Boland	John T.			
Clark	Rolla M.			
Edgington	Arthur L.			
Emmett	Edith A. (Mrs.)			
Greeno	Raphael			

Surname	Given Names	City	State	Remarks
1893 Continues				
Hough	Harry H.			
McIntosh	J. W.			
Richert	Peter			
1894				
Bell	Frank			
Dart	Jennie (Miss)			
Dunlap	Frank			
Henry	H. S.			
Matchett	John			
Parry	Fanny (Miss)			
Royer	S. L.			
1895				
Bell	Nellie (Mrs.)			Valedictorian
Boutin	Edith Clark (Mrs.)			Prize (Gold Medal)
Easly	Dora (Miss)			
Gates	W. J.			
Isaacs	Susie (Miss)			
Peet	Antoinette B. (Mrs.)			
Pottriff	Fannie L. (Mrs.)			
Spencer	Mabel (Miss)			
Starcke	Andrew H.			
Stewart	J. C.			
Todd	V. L.			
Winteer	Martha Ellis (Miss)			
1896				
Allcutt	Carrie Dickens (Miss)			
Brady	John Joseph			
Brown	Samuel J.			
Colburn	Jefferson M.			
Ellsworth	Anna Elizabeth (Miss)			
Enz	Elizabeth E. (Mrs.)			
Friesen	Julius			
Fryer	Harry M.			
Gilstrap	H. Preston			
Hancock	Avery C.			
Hancock	Mary Belle (Mrs.)			
Littlefield	Charles W.			
Miller	Robert P.			
Mills	Earnest Prudden			
Muller	Hermann Richard			
Nevitt	Rollins Roy			
Ruhl	Noah B.			
St. John	Charles H.			
Wiens	Peter			
Wise	Julius C.			

Surname	Given Names	City	State	Remarks
1897				
Andrus	Edward R.			
Antrobus	Frank B.			
Bowes	Charles C.			
Christy	Ella C. B.			
Collins	Helen M.			
Cullum	Arthur B.			
Guyer	Caroline P.			
Matzke	Samuel E.			
Putnam	Carolyn E.			
Reid	John M. (AM)			
Storry	Clark N.			
Theilmann	Emil			
Wherry	Curtis A.			
Wolff	Albert H.			
1898				
Blair	William Moore			
Browne	Herbert A.			
Clothier	Mary E.			
Cowels	John Vance			
Ditzler	Rebecca V.			
Goldman	Davilla N.			
Goodsell	Alletta			
Grant	Harrison M.			
Howell	Edwin P.			
Humphrey	John B.			
Martin	John F.			
Melcher	Fred Wilhelm			
Nolan	J. Helen			
Van Fossen	Loo B.			
1899				
Baker	E. O.	Wichita	KS	
Benthack	Peter L.	Platte City	MO	
Booth	L. R.	Valley Falls	KS	
Clothier	Samuel H.	Maple Hill	KS	
Guggenheim	L. C.	Kansas City	MO	
Lynne	Guy E. A.	Kansas City	MO	
MacLeod	D. R.	Riley	KS	
Orear	Vollerage B. "Vollie"	Kansas City	MO	
Ott	Charles W.	Kansas City	KS	

Surname	Given Names	City	State	Remarks
1900				
Benthack	Peter L.			
Brown	Amy (Mrs.)			
Collins	R. T.			
Connell	W. A. C.			
Isaacs	Elizabeth (Miss)			
Leland	William M.			
Merchers	Ferd/Fred			
Ruhl	A. M.			
Texley	Andrew			
Wilson	George H.			
1901				
Anderson	Charles Loring	Kansas City	KS	
Boyd	James Jay	Sarcoxie	MO	
Clark	Thomas J.	Centralia	MO	
McFarland	Samuel B.	Kansas City	MO	
Miller	Daniel W.	Freeman	MO	
Mooney	Belle S.	Kansas City	MO	
Nelson	George E.	Republic	KS	
Ott	Charles W., Jr.	Kansas City	MO	
Parker	Ernest E.	Oxford	IN	
Reid	Minnie Ethel	Freeman	MO	
Seymour	Sylvia	Kansas City	MO	
Smith	Derostus Elwood	Kansas City	KS	
Smith	William H.	Kansas City	KS	
1902				
Harris	Albert	Platonia	NE	
Koogler	John H.	Kansas City	MO	
Roland	Sarah Jane	Kansas City	MO	

Newspapers

03 April 1889, Young Men's Christian Association Auditorium, 1st Annual Commencement
"City News Condensed," *Kansas City (Mo.) Star,* 04 April 1889, page 1, column 4.
"Conferring the Degree of M. D.," *Kansas City (Mo.) Times,* 04 April 1889, page 2, column 2.

13 March 1890, 1213 Main Street, 2nd Annual Commencement
"A Pleasant Occasion: Commencement Exercises of the Kansas City Homeopathic Medical College," *Kansas City (Mo.) Daily Journal,* 14 March 1890, page 3, column 3.
"Homeopaths Graduated," *Kansas City (Mo.) Star,* 14 March 1890, page 1, column 2.

13 March 1891, Young Men's Christian Association Auditorium, 3rd Annual Commencement
"Six Given Diplomas: Graduates of the Kansas City Homeopathic Medical College," *Kansas City (Mo.) Daily Journal,* 14 March 1891, page 3, column 5.
"The Homoeopathic," *Kansas City (Mo.) Star,* 13 March 1891, page 3, column 3. **(no list of graduates)**

"Doctors and Dentists: Graduates of the Homeopathic and Western Dental Colleges," *Kansas City (Mo.) Star,* 14 March 1891, page 3, column 4.

"Received Their Sheepskins: Medical and Dental College Graduates Awarded Diplomas," *Kansas City (Mo.) Times,* 14 March 1891, page 5, column 1.

14 March 1892, Music Hall, 4th Annual Commencement

"Commencement Exercises: A Large Number Will Be Held during This Month," *Kansas City (Mo.) Daily Journal,* 09 March 1892, page 3, column 6. **(no list of graduates)**

"Now Write It 'M. D.,' Graduates of the Kansas City Homeopathic Medical College," *Kansas City (Mo.) Daily Journal,* 15 March 1892, page 3, columns 3-5.

"Homeopaths Graduated: Interesting Commencement Exercises at Music Hall," *Kansas City (Mo.) Star,* 15 March 1892, page 6, column 2.

15 March 1893, Coates Opera House, 5th Annual Commencement

"Ten Healers of the Sick: Graduates of the Kansas City Homeopathic Medical College," *Kansas City (Mo.) Daily Journal,* 16 March 1893, page 2, columns 2-3.

"Graduates in Medicine: Commencement Exercises of the Kansas City Homeopathic Medical College," *Kansas City (Mo.) Star,* 16 March 1893, page 7, column 5.

"Ten Brand New Doctors: Annual Commencement of the Kansas City Homeopathic Medical College," *Kansas City (Mo.) Times,* 16 March 1893, page 2, column 5.

15 March 1894, Grand Avenue Methodist Episcopal Church, 6th Annual Commencement

"Seven Graduates: Graduating Exercises of the Kansas City Homeopathic Medical College," *Kansas City (Mo.) Daily Journal,* 16 March 1894, page 3, column 6.

"Given Their Diplomas: Seven Graduates of the Kansas City Homeopathic College," *Kansas City (Mo.) Star,* 16 March 1894, page 2, column 6.

"Seven Graduates: Commencement Exercises of the Homeopathic College," *Kansas City (Mo.) Times,* 16 March 1894, page 8, column 4.

14 March 1895, Ninth Street Opera House Theater, 7th Annual Commencement

"Women in the Class: Twelve Graduates from the Kansas City Homeopathic Medical College Receive Their Diplomas," *Kansas City (Mo.) Daily Journal,* 15 March 1895, page 8, column 1.

"Homeopaths Graduating: Exercises at the College Last Night and the Commencement To-Morrow Afternoon," *Kansas City (Mo.) Star,* 13 March 1895, page 8, column 2.

"New School Doctors: The Homeopathic Medical College Graduates a Big Class," *Kansas City (Mo.) Times,* 15 March 1895, page 8, column 2.

12 March 1896, Ninth Street Opera House Theater, 8th Annual Commencement

"Twenty Graduates: The Eighth Annual Commencement Exercises of the Kansas City Homeopathic Medical College," *Kansas City (Mo.) Daily Journal,* 13 March 1896, page 8, column 2.

"Nineteen New Doctors Thursday," *Kansas City (Mo.) Star,* 09 March 1896, page 1, column 2.

"Four More Women Doctors: They Are the One-Fifth Part of the Homeopathic Class Graduated Yesterday," *Kansas City (Mo.) Star,* 13 March 1896, page 10, column 2.

"Twenty Diplomas Granted: A Score of New Graduates of the Homeopathic Medical College," *Kansas City (Mo.) Times,* 13 March 1896, page 5, column 1.

25 March 1897, Ninth Street Opera House Theater, 9th Annual Commencement

"Four Women Physicians: Kansas City Homeopathic Medical School Graduates," *Kansas City (Mo.) Daily Journal,* 26 March 1897, page 7, column 2.

"Doctors of the New School: Fourteen Disciples of Hahnemann, Four of Whom Are Women," *Kansas City (Mo.) Star,* 26 March 1897, page 4, column 1.

"Disciples of Hahnemann: Fourteen New Doctors of the New School Turned Out," *Kansas City (Mo.) Times,* 26 March 1897, page 8, column 1.

24 March 1898, Coates Opera House, 10th Annual Commencement

"Fourteen New Doctors: Ten Men and Four Women Will Graduate from the Homeopathic College Thursday," *Kansas City (Mo.) Daily Journal,* 21 March 1898, page 3, column 2. **(no list of graduates)**

"Men and Women Doctors: Fourteen Homeopathic Graduates Receive Their Deiplomas at the Coates House," *Kansas City (Mo.) Daily Journal,* 25 March 1898, page 5, column 3.

"Fourteen New Doctors: They Will Be Graduated by the Kansas City Homeopathic College Thursday," *Kansas City (Mo.) Star,* 21 March 1898, page 7, column 3. **(no list of graduates)**

"Men and Women Doctors: The Homeopathic College Gave Fourteen Their Diplomas Last Night," *Kansas City (Mo.) Star,* 25 March 1898, page 5, column 1.

"Young Doctors to Come Out: Kansas City Homeopathic Medical College Commencement," *Kansas City (Mo.) Times,* 22 March 1898, page 5, column 2.

"Complete Their Studies: Fourteen Doctors Graduated," *Kansas City (Mo.) Times,* 25 March 1898, page 5, columns 3-4.

23 March 1899, Academy of Music, 11th Annual Commencement

"Kansas City Homeopathic College," *Kansas City (Mo.) Daily Journal,* 16 March 1899, page 7, column 3.

"Two Commencements: Hahnemannian Society To-Night and Kansas City Homeopathic College Thursday Night," *Kansas City (Mo.) Daily Journal,* 21 March 1899, page 3, column 4. **(no list of graduates)**

"Nine Homeopaths: Kansas City Homeopathic Medical College Holds Its Graduating Exercises," *Kansas City (Mo.) Daily Journal,* 24 March 1899, page 5, column 5.

"Nine New Doctors: Graduated by the Kansas City Homeopathic College Last Night," *Kansas City (Mo.) Star,* 24 March 1899, page 3, column 2.

"These Are Doctors Now: Homeopathic College Holds Its Annual Commencement," *Kansas City (Mo.) Times,* 24 March 1899, page 7, column 4.

29 March 1900, Auditorium Theater, 12th Annual Commencement

"Doctors Ad Libitum: Many Commencements Arranged for This Week—Programmes Arranged," *Kansas City (Mo.) Daily Journal,* 26 March 1900, Page 10, column 3.

"Twelve New Doctors: Commencement of Kansas City Homeopathic College," *Kansas City (Mo.) Daily Journal,* 30 March 1900, page 3, column 5.

"Graduates in Homeopathy: A Class of Twelve Received Diplomas at the Auditorium To-Day," *Kansas City (Mo.) Star,* 29 March 1900, page 2, column 1.

"May Hang Out Shingles: New Homeopathic Doctors Receive Diplomas at the Auditorium," *Kansas City (Mo.) Times,* 30 March 1900, page 8, column 3.

28 March 1901, Academy of Music, 13th Annual Commencement

"Not Superstitious: Thirteen Graduates of the Homeopathic College," *Kansas City (Mo.) Daily Journal,* 29 March 1901, page 7, column 3.

"Homeopathic Graduates," *Kansas City (Mo.) Star,* 27 March 1901, page 9, column 1.

"A Graduation of Homeopaths: Ten Young Men and Three Young Women Given Diplomas Last Night," *Kansas City (Mo.) Star,* 29 March 1901, page 9, column 1.

"Have Their Diplomas Now: Nine Men and Maidens Graduate from Kansas City Homeopathic Medical College," *Kansas City (Mo.) Times,* 29 March 1901, page 5, column 1.

03 April 1902, Assembly Room of Kansas City Homeopathic College, 14th Annual Commencement

"City News in Paragraphs," *Kansas City (Mo.) Daily Journal,* 04 April 1902, page 7, column 2.

"Diplomas for Three Homeopathic Doctors," *Kansas City (Mo.) Star,* 04 April 1902, page 5, column 1.

"Its 14th Commencement: The Graduation Exercises at the Kansas City Homeopathic College," *Kansas City (Mo.) Times,* 04 April 1902, page 2, column 2.

City Directories

1886 Kansas City, Missouri, directory   —
1887 Kansas City, Missouri, directory   —
1888 Kansas City, Missouri, directory   —
1889 Kansas City, Missouri, directory   —
1890 Kansas City, Missouri, directory   —
1891 Kansas City, Missouri, directory, page 863:
    Kansas City Homoeopathic Medical College, 421 east 6th, P. Diederich, dean S. C. Delap, registrar, Mark Edgarton [sic], Treas.
1892 Kansas City, Missouri, directory, page 740:
    Kansas City Homoeopathic Medical College, 1618 Main, P. Diederich, dean, S. C. Delap, registrar, Mark Edgarton [sic], Treas.
1893 Kansas City, Missouri, directory, page 745:
    Kansas City Homoeopathic Medical College, 1022 e 10th.
1894 Kansas City, Missouri, directory, page 754:
    Kansas City Homoeopathic Medical College, 1022 e 10th.
1895 Kansas City, Missouri, directory, page 365:
    Kansas City Homoeopathic Medical College, 1022 e 10th, Dr. W D Foster dean
1896 Kansas City, Missouri, directory, page 383:
    Kansas City Homoeopathic Medical College, 1020 e 10th, W D Foster dean; W L Ray registrar
1897 Kansas City, Missouri, directory, page 887:
    Kansas City Homoeopathic Medical College, 1020 e 10th, Peter Diederich, Dean; L. G. VanScoyoc, Registrar; A. E. Neumeister, Treas.
1898 Kansas City, Missouri, directory, page 967:
    Kansas City Homoeopathic Medical College, 1020 e 10th. A. E. Neumeister, Dean; L. G. VanScoyoc, Registrar; Mark Edgerton, Treas.
1899 Kansas City, Missouri, directory, page 1084:
    Kansas City Homoeopathic Medical College, 1020 e 10th. E. E. Neumeister, Dean; L. G. VanScoyoc Registrar; Mark Edgerton Treas.
1900 Kansas City, Missouri, directory, page 1293:
    Kansas City Homoeopathic Medical College, 1020 e 10th. A. E. Neumeister, Dean; G. E. ApLynne, Registrar; Mark Edgerton Treas.
1901 Kansas City, Missouri, directory, page 581:
    Kansas City Homoeopathic Medical College 1020 e 10th H M Fryer dean, W A Connell registrar, Mark Edgerton treas
1902 Kansas City, Missouri, directory, page 627:
    Kansas City Homoeopathic Medical College 1020 e 10th S H Anderson dean, W A Connell registrar, Mark Edgerton treas

Kansas City Hospital College of Medicine
(1882-1888)

Kansas City Hospital College of Medicine was founded in 1882 and its first graduating class was in 1883. During its years of operation, twelve female physicians were graduated. This school was apparently disbanded in 1888, the year of its last known graduating class and of its last appearance in Kansas City, Missouri, directories.

Surname	Given Names	City	State	Remarks
1883				
Arnold	Rawson	Oakland	CA	
Beach	[--?--]	Olathe	KS	
Carpenter	James	Kansas City	MO	
Gilbert	James	Sibley	MO	
Granville	Edwin G.	Kansas City	MO	Valedictorian
Holman	[--?--]		MA	
Kimberlin	William H.	Kansas City	MO	
Kuchler/Knecher	Charles F.	Kansas City	MO	
Robinson	Joseph H.		TN	
1884				
Bowker	William T.	Kansas City	MO	
Breansford/Breasford	G. G.	Washington	DC	
Coombs	J. S. (Dr.)	Kansas City	MO	Ad Eundem Degree
Evans	Evan	Emporia	KS	
Fleming	J. E.	Kansas City	MO	
Kimmell	Emma J. (Mrs.)	Kansas City	MO	Valedictorian
Lieser/Tieser	Frederick D.	Cleveland	OH	
Reinhardt	George A.	Buffalo	NY	
Reinhardt	Henry M.	Buffalo	NY	
Rhodes	James (Dr.)	Boston	MA	Ad Eundem Degree
Sawyer	L. F. (Mrs.)	Kansas City	MO	
1885				
Arnold	Rawdon			
Baker	Frances A. (Mrs.)			
Beresford	Galesworth G.			
Bowker	William T.			
Carpenter	J. D.			
Chester	S. R. (Mrs.)			
Cleveland	Mary A. (Miss)			
Evans	Evan			
Fleming	John E.			
Gibbert	James			
Kimberlin	William H.			
Kimmell	Emma J. (Mrs.)			
Kuechler	Charles F.			

Surname	Given Names	City	State	Remarks
1885 Continues				
Leiser	Frederick D.			
Reinhardt	George A.			
Reinhardt	Henry M.			
Robinson	J. H.			
Rupert	L. A.			Valedictorian
Sawyer	Lucy F. (Mrs.)			
1886				
Beach	E.			
Bowker	F. P.			
Childis	M. A.			
Harris	M. E.			
Marsters	C. S.			
Newcome	E. P.			
Patty	J. H.			
Tranior/Trainor	K. B.			
1887				
Magoon	J. N.			
Merwin	D. M. G.			
Morrison	C.			
1888				
Cline	Alice B. (Miss)			Valedictorian
Cline	Permelia A. (Miss)			
Flower	Carrie B. (Miss)			
Osborne	L. S.			
Strasser	Nellie M. (Miss)			
Wilder	Annie (Miss)			
Wise	J. C.			

Newspapers

15 March 1883, Unitarian Church, 1st Annual Commencement
"Kansas City Hospital College," *Kansas City (Mo.) Daily Journal,* 16 March 1883, page 3, columns 2-3.
"Hospital College of Medicine," *Kansas City (Mo.) Times,* 16 March 1883, page 8, columns 3-4.

14 March 1884, First Baptist Church, 2nd Annual Commencement
"Hospital College Commencement," *Kansas City (Mo.) Daily Journal,* 15 March 1884, page 3, columns 1-2.
"Medical Matters," *Kansas City (Mo.) Star,* 14 March 1884, page 1, column 4. **(no list of graduates)**
"An Independent Institution: The Hospital College of Medicine Gives Its Diplomas to Nine Graduates—Strictures Up on the 'Regulars,'" *Kansas City (Mo.) Times,* 15 March 1884, page 3, column 5.

13 March 1885, College Chapel (108 West 9th Street), 3rd Annual Commencement
"Commencement Exercises," *Kansas City (Mo.) Daily Journal,* 14 March 1885, page 3, column 5. **(no list of graduates)**
"Commencement Exercises," *Kansas City (Mo.) Star,* 14 March 1885, page 2, column 2. **(no list of graduates)**

"Hospital College Graduates: Nineteen Ladies and Gentlemen Given Diplomas as Doctors—Features of the Commencement Exercises Held Last Evening," *Kansas City (Mo.) Times,* 14 March 1885, page 5, column 2.

15 March 1886, Unitarian Church, 4th Annual Commencement
"Doctors Diplomas: Graduating Exercises of the Kansas City Hospital College of Medicine," *Kansas City (Mo.) Times,* 16 March 1886, page 2, column 3.

15 Mar 1887, Chapel of the Orthopaedic Institute of the Kansas City Hospital, 5th Annual Commencement
"Hospital College of Medicine," *Kansas City (Mo.) Daily Journal,* 16 March 1887, page 4, columns 6-7.
"Twenty-Three New Doctors," *Kansas City (Mo.) Star,* 16 March 1887, page 1, column 1.
"Another Class Graduates: Diplomas Earned by Three Students of the Kansas City Hospital College of Medicine," *Kansas City (Mo.) Times,* 16 March 1887, page 8, column 3.

15 March 1888, National Business College, 6th Annual Commencement
"Medical Graduates: Commencement Exercises of the Kansas City Hospital of Medicine," *Kansas City (Mo.) Daily Journal,* 16 March 1888, page 3, column 2.
"Young Women Graduate in Medicine," *Kansas City (Mo.) Star,* 16 March 1888, page 1, column 6.
"Hospital College of Medicine," *Kansas City (Mo.) Times,* 16 March 1888, page 3, columns 3-4.

City Directories

1882 Kansas City, Missouri, directory   —
1883 Kansas City, Missouri, directory   —
1884 Kansas City, Missouri, directory, page 674:
    Kansas City Hospital College of Medicine. Main, corner Ninth. D. E. Dickerson, Dean; S. D. Bowker, Treasurer; J. Thorne, Secretary
1885 Kansas City, Missouri, directory, page 710:
    Kansas City Hospital College of Medicine. J. F. Thorne, Dean; D. E. Dickerson, Treasurer; J. D. Sherrick, Secretary.
1886 Kansas City, Missouri, directory, page 993:
    Kansas City Hospital College of Medicine. F. Coley, Dean; D. E. Dickerson, Treasurer; Griffin Reno, Secretary.
1887 Kansas City, Missouri, directory, page 821:
    Kansas City Hospital College of Medicine, F. Cooley, dean; D. E. Dickerson, treasurer; J. W. McKee, secretary, 801 Grand avenue.
1888 Kansas City, Missouri, directory, page 897:
    Kansas City Hospital College of Medicine, 19 and 20 Lockridge Hall. F. F. Cassiday, dean; E. F. Brady, secretary; A. F. Neumiester [sic], treasurer.

Kansas City Medical College
(1869-1870)

Kansas City Medical College was founded in 1869. It merged in 1870 with Kansas City College of Physicians and Surgeons (1869-1870), forming College of Physicians and Surgeons (1870-1880).

Kansas City Medical College
(1880-1905)

Kansas City Medical College, established in 1880, was formerly known as College of Physicians and Surgeons (1870-1880). Its first graduating class was in 1881. In 1905 this school merged with Medico-Chirurgical College (1898-1905) and College of Physicians and Surgeons of the Kansas City [KS] University (1894-1905), forming School of Medicine of the University of Kansas (1905-).

Surname	Given Names	City	State	Remarks
1881				
Beeson	Edward T.	Spring Hill	KS	
Fay	William M.	Denver	CO	
Foster	Harvey A.	Ottawa	KS	Prize ($25)
Hardin	Charles B.	Independence	MO	
Knoche	J. Phillip	Kansas City	MO	
Knox	Marshall D.	Milford	TX	
Lewis	Alfred	Tecumseh	NE	
McHenry	James	Minneapolis	KS	
Phillips	John M.	Lawrence	KS	
Randall	Maxin	Kansas City	MO	Prize ($100), Valedictorian
Winfrey	N. B.	Pleasant Hill	MO	
Woodul	James H.	Kansas City	MO	
1882				
Baldwin	F. V.	Modoc	MO	
Bayliss	William M.	Aubrey	KS	Prize (Book), Valedictorian
Bradford	C. B.	Council Grove	KS	
Dartt	C. N.	Kansas City	MO	
Elwood	Frank B.	Beatrice	NE	Prize ($25)
Griffith	D. R.	Rose Hill	MO	
Logan	J. B.	Kansas City	MO	
McIlvain	J. R.	Council Grove	KS	
Overstreet	J. A.	Emporia	KS	2 Prizes (Instruments & Book)
Puderbaugh	A.	Osawkie	KS	
Reddish	W. T.	Barry	MO	
Simpson	William J.	Waldron	MO	2 Prizes ($100, Book)
Slaughter	R. F.	Aubrey	KS	
Stolte	L. C.	Franklin Center	IA	
Sturgis	John	Wawaka	IN	
True	G. P.	Douglass	KS	

Surname	Given Names	City	State	Remarks
1883				
Ball	Henry P.	Shawnee	KS	
Chambliss	Charles M.	Bozeman	MT Territory	
Coates	Samuel R.	Kansas City	MO	Prize ($25)
Fisher	Joseph S.	Middleport	OH	
Griffith	Charles E.	Rose Hill	MO	
Ironsides	Alexander H.	Kansas City	MO	Prize (Book)
Ladd	James R.	Cambridge	MO	
Phillips	Edwin T.	Manhattan	KS	Prize ($100)
Pitcher	Henry E.	Shawnee Mound	MO	
Walker	Richard P.	Platte City	MO	Prize (Instruments)
Wann	John B.	Harisonville	MO	
Young	William H.	Springdale	AR	
1884				
Barraclough	A. W.	Kansas City	MO	
Basham	D. W.	San Marcus	TX	
Bernhardt	Chris C.	Wyandotte	KS	
Dudley	W. S.	Thayer	KS	
Eager	J. L./S. B.	Wyandotte	KS	
Janeway	D. F.	Malvern	KS	
Lewis	P. M.	Lecompton	KS	
Main	G. W.	Monroe	MO	
Overholzer	M. P.	Horner	KS	
Pettijohn/Pettyjohn	N. J.	Hot Springs	NM	
Singleton	G. M.	Kansas City	MO	
Sloan	R. T.	Kansas City	MO	
Stowers	I./J. P.	Holt	MO	
Surber	C. C.	Perry	KS	
Yows/Yorns	J. M.	Centertown	MO	
1885				
Adair	Thomas W.	Adrian/ Adrain	MO	
Beattie	Thomas J.	Kansas City	MO	Prize ($35)
Burnett	Steven D.	Council Grove	KS	
Cresap	Roger N.	Kansas City	MO	Prize ($100)
Holliway	C. L.	Kansas City	MO	
Hutchison	Robert C.	Olathe	KS	
Miller	Isaac M.	Montrose	MO	Prize (Instruments)
Sumner	Charles O.	Kansas City	MO	
Wahl	Edward D.	Abilene	KS	Prizes (Instruments & Books)

Surname	Given Names	City	State	Remarks
1886				
Atchison	James R./B.			
Diffenderfer	J. W.			
Guinn	James R.			
Horner	Levi			
Miller	James M.			
Moore	Edwin T.			
Schenck	A. W.			
Smith	Budd			Prize ($25)
Torrance/Torrens	Wiliam			Prize (Instruments)
Wright	George E./G.			2 Prizes ($100 & Book)
1887				
Barber	William David			
Barker	John F.			
Broyles	Franklin Hunt			
Connell	Joseph B.			Prize ($100)
Day	John O.			
Fay	Joseph Ransom			
Ferguson	Wilson Jones			
Herrington	Sterling Price			
Hull	John Crawford			
Langworthy	Simon Burton			Prize ($25)
Lee	William Henry			
Scott	Frank Marion			
1888				
Boggs	J. D./R.			
Bowling	J. A.			
Buzick/Busic	E.			
Cox	T. A.			
Crawford	W. E.			
Dunkeson/Dunkerson	W. L.			Prize ($100)
Frick	W. J.			Prize
Koepsel	R. L.			
Marks	M. F.			Prize
Marshall	J. E.			
McGill	J. F.			
McVey	W. E.			
Michael	W. L.			
Moore	T. B.			
Patton	C. W.			
Rankin	E. C.			
Sumner/Simmer	G. L.			
Traylor	J. B.			
Walker	J. D.			
Winn	J. W.			2 Prizes ($25 & Instruments)

Surname	Given Names	City	State	Remarks
1889				
Benton	William Henry			
Cross	Robert Orr			Prize ($25)
Davis	Thomas Orville			
Duckett	Thomas Henry			
Goss	George Washington			
Herndon	Albert Sidney			
Hodges	William Henry			
Lambeth	George Benjamin			
Logan	James Nelson			
Mahr	John Charles			
Marsh	Will Q.			
Martin	George Samuel			Prize (Book)
Mauser	William Henry			
Musgrove	Robert Green			
Tullis	John Wheeler			
Van Tuyl	William Russell			Prize ($100)
Wherrell	John			
Wilson	Charles Edgar			
1890				
Anderson	F. L.			
Bacon	C. B./E.			
Elliott	J. M.			
Fryer	J. L.			Prize (Book)
Himoe	H. C.			
Holmes	A. T.			
Johnson	J. H./W.			
Krueger	O. W.			
Linderman	Edgar			
Lowman	R. C.			Prize ($100)
McFarland	W. L.			
McGee	R. L./S.			Prize ($25)
O'Neil	A. A.			
Parker	P. B.			
Petty	G. W.			
Thrailkill/Threilkill	E. H.			Prize (Instruments)
1891				
Bullock	Edward R.	Kansas City	MO	
Carney	Ira	Clinton	MO	
Cheney	Enos R.	McPherson	KS	Prize ($25)
Clements	Joseph C.	Kansas City	MO	
DeMay	W. A.	Cedar Bluffs	KS	
Florey	Orville H.	St. Edwards	NE	
Fulkerson	Walter/William C.	Cumberland Gap	VA	
Griffith	Joseph K.	Clayton	MO	
Harden	Charles R.	El Dorado	KS	

Surname	Given Names	City	State	Remarks
1891 Continues				
Jones	James E.	Kansas City	MO	
Lewers	Frederick K.	Kansas City	MO	
McCall	Horace B.	Kansas City	MO	
Pontius	Calvin E.	Akron	IN	Prize (Book)
Slagle	Marion/Morris E.	Slagle	MO	
Sloan	John R.	Stanley	KS	
Smith	George S.	Liberal	KS	
Strawn	Joel N.	Shilloway / Shallaway	KS	
Stubbs	Charles L.	Chicago	IL	Prize (Book)
Sweeney	Charles T.	Warrensburg	MO	Prize ($100)
Thrush	Thomas B.	Cameron	MO	Prize (Instruments)
Truex	James L.	Denver	CO	
Underwood	Johnson	Kansas City	MO	
1892				
Brewer	William Philip			
Cadwell	Victor			
Carnahan	Joseph Lynn			
Cloud	Marshal Morgan			Prize ($25)
Coffin	George Oliver			
Cornell	Howard Merritt			
Crosswhite	John Webster			
Doggett	Elmer Ellsworth			
Fulkerson	Emmett Wentworth			
Haynes	Lorenzo Dow			
Kindred	Homer Leander			
Lawson	Oscar Sutton			
Lee	James Grant			
Lyon	James Ira			
Messer	George Frederick			
Miller	James Harley			
Morrrow	James William			
Murdock	Fred Judson			
Murphy	Franklin Edward			Prize (Book)
Ozias	Charles Othello			
Perry	Elmer Ellsworth			
Pike	Columbus Jefferson			
Read	John William			
Roberts	James Linsey			
Robinson	Losson Roisencrans			
Robinson	Oliver Theron			
Rowe	Drury Bridgeman			
Sawyer	Lewis Berdine			
Shuck	Lee Irvine			
Stevens	Thomas Andrew			

Surname	Given Names	City	State	Remarks
1892 Continues				
Taylor	Trueman Elsworth			
Thomas	William Sherman			
Vaughan	James Alexander			
Wellman	Fred Craton			Prize ($100)
1893				
Bell	R. M.			
Bell	William M.			
Blake	John H.			
Calnan	George B.			
Canfield	Herbert H.			Prize
Coffey	George W.			Prize
Dunkeson	Edward B.			
Frick	Charles B.			Prize
Gates	Charles O.			
Gray	James M.			Prize ($25)
Johnson	Grant T.			
Lattridge	Melome H.			
McArthur	John F.			
Murdock	Samuel			
Noon	Nicholas R.			
Vaughan	William F.			
Yates	William S.			Prize ($100)
1894				
Beedle	Gordon Augustus	Kansas City	MO	
Bollinger	Howard Elmus	Everest	KS	
Bower	Willis Brickley	Lenexa	KS	
Brunig	Fred H. (Ph. G.)	Kansas City	MO	Prize ($25)
Chambliss	Edward Lawrence	Kansas City	MO	Prizes;Book, Instruments
Cossins	William Truman	Bolivar	MO	
Cranston	Charles Oscar	Parsons	KS	
Duvall	Hunter Jesse	Abbeyville	KS	
Ellis	James M.	Kansas City	MO	
Fields	Tom	Lee's Summit	MO	
Finnegan	John Thomas	Kansas City	MO	
Harrelson	Nathan O.	Kansas City	MO	
Hashinger	George Henry (PhG)	Kansas City	MO	
Huffaker	Duke Hunter	Westport	MO	
Keller	Robert Graham	Pleasant Hill	MO	
Kernodle	James D.	Kansas City	MO	
Kirkpatrick	Andrew M.	Blue Mound	KS	
Kirkpatrick	Joseph Spellman	Blue Mound	KS	
Kreeger	Charles Lucien	Cockrell	MO	
Millikan	Solomon J.	Pittsburg	MO	
Neptune	John W.	Elmo	KS	

Surname	Given Names	City	State	Remarks
1894 Continues				
Otterman	James Lewis	Kansas City	MO	
Overall	Thomas Wilson	Kansas City	MO	Prize
Ragan	Stephen Hood	Kansas City	MO	
Rees	John Thomas	Florence	KS	
Robertson	John Theophilus	Bolivar	TN	
Schaeffer	Leo Alonzo	Kansas City	MO	Prize
Smith	Andrew Jackson (PhG)	Leavenworth	KS	Prize ($100)
Stephens	John Morse	Clinton	MO	
Thomas	Olin Carl	Olathe	KS	
Watts	Robert B.	Kansas City	MO	
Wheeler	Bertan Henry	Westport	MO	
Wood	Henry Lee	Napa City	CA	
1895				
Alch	George Harris			
Armour	Wallace A.			
Beem	Edward David			
Bennett	Gerritt Judd			
Bowers	Horace Sanford			
Chambers	Harry Leslie			2 Prizes ($100)
Chandler	John Franklin			Prize (Book)
Clarke	Samuel Columbus			
Cooke	William Fleetwood			
Corns	Charles Vaile			
Harbaugh	Charles Carleton			
Hill	Howard			Prize ($25)
Hughes	John Henry			
Kitchen	John Chapel			Prize (Instruments)
Kreeger	George G.			
Krueger	Ernest Adolph			
Paddock	Edward Everett			
Peugh	Edwin DeWayn			
Rowland	J. Walter			
Sharp	Orlan Dayton			
Tesson	Noah Albert Grant			
Towers	George Nelson			
Wall	Arthur Harvey			
Watson	B. Frank			
Way	Franklin Eliada			
West	Charles Owen			
White	William Thomas			
1896				
Amyx	John S.	Merwin	MO	
Barber	Oliver S.	Kansas City	MO	
Burns	Lee M. (PhG)	Kansas City	MO	
Cable	Colin	Kansas City	KS	

Surname	Given Names	City	State	Remarks
1896 Continues				
Crabtree	John W.	Johnstown	MO	
Dailey	Forrest W.	Higginsville	MO	Prize (Instruments)
Ebright	Edwin D.	Marion	KS	Prize (Book)
George	John H.	Kansas City	MO	
Hawley	Harry L.	Valley Falls	KS	
Helwig	Orville H.	Kansas City	KS	
Hobbs	Arthur A.	Kansas City	MO	
Hornback	Joseph T.	Sprague	MO	
Ingles	Anson B.	Larned	KS	
Joy	Andrew O'C.	Nevada	MO	
Maloney	Harry W. (PhG)	Shawnee	KS	
McKinney	Kirk C. (BA)	Kansas City	MO	
Miller	John W. (PhG)	Kansas City	KS	Prize (Instruments)
Miller	William A.	Perham	MN	
Petty	Charles N.	Ransom	KS	
Riddell	John DeW. (BS)	Conway	KS	
Sams	William M. (LB)	Kansas City	MO	Prize ($25)
Shenck	Samuel K. (MDC)	Salina	KS	
Simonton	Edgar L.	Louisville	KS	
Skinner	Benjamin (BS)	Fairview	KS	Prize ($100)
Smith	Delmar H.	Paola	KS	Prize (Instruments)
Steadman	John R.	Waddill	KS	
Steele	Samuel	Phoenix	AZ Territory	
Ward	Thomas J.	Birmingham	MO	
Young	Oscar O.	East Lynne	MO	
1897				
Allen	J. G.	Hatfield	MO	
Allen	William H., Jr.	Rich Hill	MO	
Boeber	E. Julius, Jr.	Westport	MO	
Botts	William F. (BS)	Kansas City	MO	
Campbell	W. L.	Kansas City	MO	
Courtney	Charles F. (BS)	Springdale	KS	
Crooks	O. R.	Kansas City	MO	
Dougan	Archie L.	Asheboro	NC	
Green	John V.	Kansas City	MO	
Henderson	William R.	Oak Grove	MO	
Heylmun	Harry	Kansas City	MO	3 Prizes
Jacobs	Benjamin (LLB)	Lawrence	KS	
Jones	Walter K.	Kansas City	MO	
Lee	Loren E.	Winston	MO	
Massey	Thomas E. (PB)	Holt	MO	
Miller	Hugh (BL)	Doniphan	KS	
Netherton	George T. (MDC)	Gallatin	MO	
Parker	Orrin H. (PhG)	Arkansas City	KS	
Paul	J. B. (PhG)	Kansas City	MO	
Peck	Nelson E.	Kansas City	MO	

Surname	Given Names	City	State	Remarks
1897 Continues				
Phillips	Dalton L.	Hicks City	MO	
Ragsdale	James H.	Smith Center	KS	
Ralph	Benjamin B.	Red Lake Falls	MN	Prize ($50)
Rhoades	Herbert A.	Sprague	MO	Prize ($25)
Sawyer	James F.	Kansas City	MO	
Saylor	Harvey W.	Morrill	KS	
Slaughter	Charles V.	Olathe	KS	
Smith	Arthur M. (PhG)	Moline	KS	
Smith	Harry P.	Kingsville	MO	
Soden	Frank J. (PhG)	Kansas City	MO	
Sturgis	Wylie E. (PB)	Perrin	MO	
Talbott	Albert S.	Kansas City	MO	
Van Eman	Frederick T.	Kansas City	MO	Prize ($50)
Wilson	William P.	Westmoreland	KS	Prize (Instruments)
1898				
Alton	Glover P.	Sedalia	MO	
Blasdel	Giles A.	Plevna	KS	
Bostick	Will	Holden	MO	
Bowline	Benjamin F.	Zebra	MO	
Braecklein	Oscar R.	Kansas City	MO	
Brown	Albert L.	Leavenworth	KS	2 Prizes (Instruments)
Brunig	Henry	Kansas City	MO	
Campbell	Samuel T.	Clarkson	OK Territory	
Carter	John W.	Kansas City	MO	
Cheney	James W.	McPherson	KS	Prize ($100)
Clarke	Howard L.	Olathe	KS	
Collins	Davis W.	Wellsville	KS	
Dalby	Phillip J.	Sedan	KS	
Davis	J. Frank	Wellsville	KS	
Dickinson	Rollin J.	Kirwin	KS	
Fuller	James S.	Fort Gibson	Indian Territory	
Gaines	Edgar F.	Bates City	MO	
Gracieux	Ph. J.	Kansas City	MO	
Kaull	Lee P.	Beloit	KS	Prize (Instruments)
Kennedy	Samuel G.	Tulsa	Indian Territory	
Kirkpatrick	Charles E.	Blue Mound	KS	
Koons	Franklin W.	Alden	KS	
Longacre	Charles E.	Pleasant Hill	MO	
Martin	Harry	Kansas City	MO	
Matthews	Frank L.	Joplin	MO	
McBride	Joseph S.	Conway	KS	
Means	William G.	Kansas City	KS	
Monahan	James H.	Kansas City	MO	
Nichols	Herman V.	Manhattan	KS	
Norman	William G.	Logan	IA	Prize ($25)

Surname	Given Names	City	State	Remarks
1898 Continues				
O'Flaherty	Aloysius E.	Kansas City	MO	
Pallett	William H.	Crete	NE	
Palmer	William R.	Kansas City	KS	
Pickard	Matthew W.	Kansas City	MO	
Pinkston	Omar W.	Kansas City	MO	
Reed	J. Frank	Kansas City	MO	
Reynolds	John W.	Creston	IA	
Shockley	Major Augustus W.	Leavenworth	KS	2 Prizes (Book)
Thacker	R. Emmett (MD)	Bradley	Indian Territory	
Thume	George W.	Kansas City	MO	
Van Blarcom	Samuel L.	Kansas City	KS	
1899				
Bockhorst	Arthur L.	Milwaukee	WI	
Branaman	Abraham	Kansas City	MO	
Byram	Wiliam M.	Richmond	MO	
Campbell	George C.	Clarkson	OK	
Carbaugh	Eugene	Kansas City	MO	
Carson	Robert T.	Kansas City	MO	
Chambers	Albert M.	Talihina	Indian Territory	
Coberly	Lee J.	Concordia	KS	
Davis	Arthur E.	Sulphur Springs	TX	
Duff	Talbot S.	Princeton	MO	
Emerson	Burr H.	Bolivar	MO	
Evans	Charles W.	Larned	KS	Prize
Ferguson	Ray	Wellington	KS	2 Prizes ($25)
Grisell	William S.	Bartley	NE	
Grosshart	Ross	Creighton	MO	
Hazen	Abraham L.	Sabetha	KS	
Henderson	Ralph C.	Erie	KS	Prize
Hueyette	H. Perrie	Kansas City	MO	
Kelley	Eugene H.	Odessa	MO	
Knox	Andrew C.	Independence	MO	Prize (Book)
Lester	Will H.	Greenville	MI	
Longnecker	Charles W.	Paola	KS	
Longnecker	Oscar M.	Paola	KS	
Martin	J. Ross	Hume	MO	
Randall	Frank W.	Leavenworth	MO	2 Prizes ($100)
Sheridan	Allen V.	Paola	KS	
Stapp	Joseph H.	Morton	MO	
Stepp	J. Edward	Lancaster	KS	
Tonge	James A. G.	Hume	MO	
Van Allen	John P.	Kirwin	KS	

1900

Barker/Baker	Robert E.	WV	
Black	Guy H.	KS	
Boyer	Edward J.	MO	
Boyle	John M.	KS	
Clark	Zachary J.	OK	
Clutz/Klutz	Ralph R.	KS	
Colvin	Charles H.	MO	
Dennis	Adolphus J.	MO	
Evans	John H.	UT	
Fannin	Frank A.	AR	
Felch	Harvey J.	WA	
Fisher	Charles M.	KS	
Fitzgerald	Dennie L.	NE	
Frizzell	James T.	MO	
Gilham	Ernest M.	MO	
Grove	Bennie E.	OK	
Hall	Frank J.	MO	
Harris	Louis A.	CA	
Harvey	Robert J.	KS	
Hedrick	Clement L. V.	MO	
Henderson	Robert G.	NE	
Hibbard	James S.	KS	Prize ($25)
Jack	William G.	KS	
Kussart	Jacob G.	IA	
Lee	Frank W.	NE	
Little	William H.	KS	
Maguire	Edward	WA	
McCarty	Charles W.	KS	
McPherson	Owen P.	KS	
McVicker	William D.	KS	
Murray	David J.	MO	
Nicholson	George M.	CT	
Reitzel	Walter M.	KS	
Revell	Arthur F.	KS	
Sharon	Franklin F.	MO	Prize ($100)
Sherry	Laban C.	MO	
Shy	Milton P.	MO	Prize
Speer	Newton C.	KS	Prize (Book)
Stahlman	David C.	KS	
Stout	Frank B.	KS	Prize (Instruments)
Stowers	Guy A.	MO	
Taggart	Henry H.	KS	
Thompson	Claude A.	Indian Territory	
Tinney	Charles M.	KS	
Toothaker	Benjamin W.	KS	Prize (Instruments)
Trimble	William K.	MO	
Vanniman/Vaniman	Jesse W.	KS	
Wortman	Jacob G.	KS	
Young	Frank B.	AR	

Surname	Given Names	City	State	Remarks
1901				
Bonham	James M./N.			Prize ($25)
Goldman	Max			Prize ($100)
Griffith	J. G.			Prize (Instruments)
Koons	Clayton C.			Prize (Instruments)
McCall	Pearl C.			Prize (Instruments)
Wellman	Clarence L.			Prize
Also 39 others				
1902				
Adams	Charles F.			
Barber	Charles M.			2 Prizes (Instruments)
Bentz	George H.			2 Prizes
Breese	Harry E.			
Castelaw	Rush E.			
Crawford	Harry S.			
Davis	Albert W.			Prize ($100)
Gainey	J. H.			
Hutchison/Hutchins	T. L.			
Lee	Clarence E.			
Longnecker	George W.			Prize ($25)
Manson	David W.			
Peairs	J. E.			
Skaife	Robert J.			
Smith	Robert M.			
Turner	A. J.			
Wachter	Egon			
White	Warren E.			
Witman	Paul B./P.			
1903				
Albers	Edward August			Prize (Instruments)
Barney	Louie Frank			Prize ($25)
Beshoar	Benjamin B.			
Bird	Arthur A.			
Brunig	Conrad P.			
Brunner	Benjamin			
Burnett	Edward J.			
Carlton	Arthur L.			
Faulkner	James Thomas			Prize ($100)
Ferguson	Robert L.			
Gilliland	Alvin O.			
Ginsberg	Edward L.			
Hanna	Minford Armour			Prize (Instruments)

Surname	Given Names	City	State	Remarks
1903 Continues				
Hinshaw	Jonathan D.			
Jackson	Robert S.			
Lambers	Wesley F.			
Pickerill	George Reynolds			Prize
Smith	Rheuben C.			
Stewart	Edward Lovelle			2 Prizes (Book)
Tinney	Ray M.			
Toothaker	Sylvester R.			
Townsdin	Asa M.			
Vittum	James S.			
West	William C.			
1904				
Abrams	William E.			Prize
Adams	Alonzo R.			
Albright	William E.			
Bertholf	Charles M.			Prize
Blake	Frank R.			
Brentlinger	Leland G.			
Brumm	William E.			
Buhler	David B.			
Carrnrae	Lewis, Jr.			
Carter	William H.			Prize
Daughters	Heaton G.			
Edgerton	Harry Walton			Prize ($25)
Ewing	Henry Z.			
Gimler	Herman E.			
Hershner	Charles S.			
Holbrook	Ralph W.			
Johnson	Franklin T.			
Lambdin	Hiram S.			Prize
McKittrick	Charles E.			
Milne	Louis A.			
Mollison	Joseph A.			
Neel	William H.			
Nichols	Walter J.			
Powers	John Harold			Prize ($100)
Richardson	William			
Saylor	John H.			
Shelton	Frank W.			
Smith	Thomas E.			Prize
Taggart	Frank B.			
Trueheart	Marion			

Surname	Given Names	City	State	Remarks
1904 Continues				
Wallace	Floyd E.			
Wilson	Walter L.			
Wright	Ozra			
Wyatt	Douglas, Jr.			
1905				
Abrams	Corydon Jackson			Prize
Blades	Joseph Brewer			
Boyd	George Thomas			
Brewster	Roger B.			
Campbell	Isaac A.			
Carson	L. Russell			
Cole	Hugh Hamilton			
Cook	Laurence C.			
Doms	Henry C. A.			
Edgerton	Sol Meredith			
Faires	Oliver Perry			Prize
Florian	Albert J.			Prize ($100)
Harvey	Fredric E.			
Helman	Claude H.			
Huddle	William I.			
Hudiburg	Walter S.			
Hull	Ralph W.			
Jones	Zachariah G.			
Lambdin	J. D. Moore			
Mahoney	James T.			
Miller	Charles M.			
Moennighoff	Fritz J.			Prize (Instruments)
Neighbors	Clarence A.			
Ray	James Edwin			
Robertson	Wright			
Russell	R. Lee			
Sherfey	James William			2 Prizes ($25)
Smith	C. Nelson			Prize
Smith	Norris A.			
Thomas	Clifton Allen			
Tipton	F. Earl			
Tretbar	Friedrich W.			
Walker	Homer Moss			
Wittwer	Edward C.			

Newspapers

01 March 1881, Central Presbyterian Church (South), 12th Annual Commencement
"A Dozen More: New Physicians Sent Forth by the Kansas City Medical College," *Kansas City (Mo.) Daily Journal,* 02 March 1881, page 5, columns 3-4.
"Making More Medics: Commencement Exercises of the Kansas City Medical College, To-Night," *Kansas City (Mo.) Star,* 01 March 1881, page 1, column 1.
"Doctors' Degrees: Annual Commencement of the Kansas City Medical College," *Kansas City (Mo.) Times,* 02 March 1881, page 5, column 1.

07 March 1882, Walnut Street Methodist Episcopal Church (South), 13th Annual Commencement
"The Thirteenth Annual Commencement of the Kansas City Medical College: Interesting Exercises Connected with the Graduation of Sixteen Students—The Address," *Kansas City (Mo.) Daily Journal,* 08 March 1882, page 4, columns 5-6, page 5, columns 1-3.
"More M. D.'s: Graduating Exercises of the Kansas City Medical College," *Kansas City (Mo.) Star,* 08 March 1882, page 4, column 2.
"More Graduates: Commencement Exercises of the Kansas City Medical College Tuesday Night," *Kansas City (Mo.) Times,* 05 March 1882, page 6, column 3.
"Men of Medicine: Graduation Exercises at the Kansas City Medical College," *Kansas City (Mo.) Times,* 08 March 1882, page 8, columns 1-6, page 5, columns 5-6.

06 March 1883, Walnut Street Methodist Episcopal Church (South), 14th Annual Commencement
"Commencement: Fourteenth Annual Graduation Exercises of the Kansas City Medical College—Addresses and Banquet," *Kansas City (Mo.) Daily Journal,* 07 March 1883, page 3, columns 1-3.
"Doctors Dine: The Commencement Exercises and Banquet Last Night," *Kansas City (Mo.) Star,* 07 March 1883, page 1, column 4.
"Medical College Commencement," *Kansas City (Mo.) Times,* 07 March 1883, page 8, columns 1-2.

04 March 1884, Coates Opera House, 15th Annual Commencement
"'Healers,' Fifteenth Annual Commencement of the Kansas City Medical College," *Kansas City (Mo.) Daily Journal,* 05 March 1884, page 5, columns 1-5.
"Annual Commencement," *Kansas City (Mo.) Star,* 03 March 1884, page 1, column 3. **(no list of graduates)**
"Sixteen New Doctors: Fifteenth Annual Commencement of the Kansas City College of Medicine—The Exercises and the Banquet," *Kansas City (Mo.) Times,* 05 March 1884, page 8, column 1.

17 March 1885, First Baptist Church, 16th Annual Commencement
"Medical and Dental Graduates," *Kansas City (Mo.) Daily Journal,* 18 March 1885, page 3, columns 2-3.
"Commencement Exercises," *Kansas City (Mo.) Star,* 18 March 1885, page 2, column 4. **(no list of graduates)**
"Fifteenth Commencement: Graduating Exercises of the Kansas City Medical and Dental Colleges—Prizes Conferred," *Kansas City (Mo.) Times,* 18 March 1885, page 8, column 3.

16 March 1886, Music Hall, 17th Annual Commencement
"More Doctors of Medicine," *Kansas City (Mo.) Daily Journal,* 17 March 1886, page 3, columns 1-2.
"Diplomas Awarded," *Kansas City (Mo.) Star,* 17 March 1886, page 1, column 7. **(no list of graduates)**
"Twelve New Doctors: Graduating Exercises of the Kansas City Medical College—Diplomas Awarded," *Kansas City (Mo.) Times,* 17 March 1886, page 8, column 2.
"Twelve New Doctors: Graduating Exercises of the Kansas City Medical College—Diplomas Awarded," *Kansas City (Mo.) Times,* 17 March 1886, page 8, column 2.

15 March 1887, Music Hall, 18th Annual Commencement
"College Commencement: Graduating Exercises of Two Kansas City Medical Institutions—Addresses Delivered," *Kansas City (Mo.) Daily Journal,* 16 March 1887, page 4, columns 5-7.
"Twenty-Three New Doctors," *Kansas City (Mo.) Star,* 16 March 1887, page 1, column 1.
"Kansas City Medical Association," *Kansas City (Mo.) Times,* 16 March 1887, page 8, column 3.

13 March 1888, Music Hall, 19th Annual Commencement
"Commencement Exercises: Graduates in Medicine and Dentistry Receive Their Diplomas—An Address by Rev. Cameron Mann," *Kansas City (Mo.) Daily Journal,* 14 March 1888, page 3, columns 1-2.
"Doctors' Degrees: Graduation Exercises of the Kansas City Medical and Dental Colleges," *Kansas City (Mo.) Times,* 14 March 1888, page 8, column 3.

11 March 1889, Music Hall, 20th Annual Commencement
"Coming Events," *Kansas City (Mo.) Star,* 05 March 1889, page 1, column 4. **(no list of graduates)**
"The Twentieth Annual," *Kansas City (Mo.) Star,* 11 March 1889, page 2, column 7. **(no list of graduates)**
"New Doctors and Dentists," *Kansas City (Mo.) Star,* 12 March 1889, page 1, column 2. **(no list of graduates)**
"Doctors and Dentists: Commencement Exercises of the Colleges of Medicine and Dental Surgery," *Kansas City (Mo.) Times,* 12 March 1889, page 2, column 3.

10 March 1890, Young Men's Christian Association Hall, 21st Annual Commencement
"Received Their Diplomas: An Addition of Sixteen to the Medical Profession," *Kansas City (Mo.) Daily Journal,* 11 March 1890, page 8, columns 1-3.
"Knights of Scalpel and Pill: The Kansas City Medical College Graduates Sixteen Young Men," *Kansas City (Mo.) Star,* 08 March 1890, page 6, column 3.
"Doctors Banquet: Twenty-First Anniversary of the Kansas City Medical College Celebrated," *Kansas City (Mo.) Times,* 11 March 1890, page 5, column 4. **(no list of graduates)**

16 March 1891, Music Hall, 22nd Annual Commencement
"Degrees and Prizes: Commencement Exercises of the Kansas City Medical College," *Kansas City (Mo.) Daily Journal,* 17 March 1891, page 3, columns 1-2.
"The Kansas City Medical: The Oldest Institution in the City—Commencement Exercises," *Kansas City (Mo.) Star,* 13 March 1891, page 3, column 3.
"Are Young Esculapians Now: Twenty-Second Commencement of the Kansas City Medical College," *Kansas City (Mo.) Times,* 17 March 1891, page 2, column 6.

15 March 1892, Music Hall, 23rd Annual Commencement
"Commencement Exercises: A Large Number Will Be Held during This Month," *Kansas City (Mo.) Daily Journal,* 09 March 1892, page 3, column 6. **(no list of graduates)**
"Ready for Patients: The Kansas City Medical College Confers Degrees upon Graduates," *Kansas City (Mo.) Daily Journal,* 16 March 1892, page 7, column 1.
"Doctors of Medicine: The Degree Conferred upon Thirty-Four Graduates Last Night," *Kansas City (Mo.) Star,* 16 March 1892, page 6, column 2.
"Will Battle with Disease: Thirty-Four Eager Recruits for the Army of Physicians," *Kansas City (Mo.) Times,* 16 March 1892, page 8, column 3.

20 March 1893, Music Hall, 24th Annual Commencement
"Young Physicians: Seventeen Graduates of the Kansas City Medical College Given Diplomas," *Kansas City (Mo.) Daily Journal,* 21 March 1893, page 3, column 2. **(no list of graduates)**
"Their College Days Over: Graduates of the Kansas City Medical College Receive Diplomas," *Kansas City (Mo.) Star,* 21 March 1893, page 6, column 2.
"Seventeen More Doctors: Commencement Exercises of the Kansas City Medical College," *Kansas City (Mo.) Times,* 21 March 1893, page 2, columns 1-2.

22 March 1894, Coates Opera House, 25th Annual Commencement
"Ready for a Call: Thirty-One Young Physicians Receive Their diplomas and Will Return Home Happy," *Kansas City (Mo.) Daily Journal,* 23 March 1894, page 3, column 4. **(no list of graduates)**
"Thirty-Two New Doctors: Twenty-Fifth Commencement of the Kansas City Medical College," *Kansas City (Mo.) Star,* 20 March 1894, page 3, column 3.
"Thirty-One New Physicians: Commencement Exercises of the Kansas City Medical College," *Kansas City (Mo.) Times,* 23 March 1894, page 8, columns 1-3.

26 March 1895, Auditorium Theater, 26th Annual Commencement

"Twenty-Seven Graduates: The Twenty-Sixth Annual Commencement of the Kansas City Medical College—Alumni Banquet," *Kansas City (Mo.) Daily Journal,* 27 March 1895, page 3, column 4.

"Medical Students Graduating: The Kansas City Medical College to Give Diplomas to Twenty-Eight To-Night," *Kansas City (Mo.) Star,* 26 March 1895, page 8, column 2.

"Students Become Doctors: Annual Commencement of the Kansas City Medical College—Winners of Prizes," *Kansas City (Mo.) Star,* 27 March 1895, page 8, column 3.

"To Rescue the Perishing: That Is What Twenty-Seven Young Men Expect to Do," *Kansas City (Mo.) Times,* 27 March 1895, page 5, column 3.

26 March 1896, Auditorium Theater, 27th Annual Commencement

"They Are Now Physicians: Commencement of the Kansas City Medical College," *Kansas City (Mo.) Daily Journal,* 27 March 1896, page 8, column 1.

"Twenty-Nine New Doctors: Commencement Exercises of the Kansas City Medical College To-Night," *Kansas City (Mo.) Star,* 26 March 1896, page 8, column 3.

"New Doctors and Old Ones: Commencement and Alumni Meeting of Kansas City Medical College," *Kansas City (Mo.) Times,* 27 March 1896, page 8, column 3.

29 March 1897, Coates Opera House, 28th Annual Commencement

"They Are Doctors Now: Kansas City Medical College Graduates 34 Students," *Kansas City (Mo.) Daily Journal,* 30 March 1897, page 3, column 5.

"More New Doctors: Thirty-Four Will Graduate from the Kansas City Medical College Monday," *Kansas City (Mo.) Star,* 27 March 1897, page 8, column 1.

"More Doctors Graduated: The Kansas City Medical College Commencement Exercises with 34 Graduates," *Kansas City (Mo.) Star,* 30 March 1897, page 8, column 2.

"Ready to Cure the Sick: Thirty-Four Young Doctors Are Given Their Degrees," *Kansas City (Mo.) Times,* 30 March 1897, page 2, column 1.

21 March 1898, Coates Opera House, 29th Annual Commencement

"Reach the Top by Degrees: Forty Graduated from Kansas City Medical College," *Kansas City (Mo.) Daily Journal,* 22 March 1898, page 3, column 1.

"They are 'M D's' Now: The Kansas City Medical College Graduates Forty-One New Doctors," *Kansas City (Mo.) Star,* 22 March 1898, page 7, column 4.

"May Hang Out Shingles Now: Forty-One Doctors Are Turned Out by a Medical School," *Kansas City (Mo.) Times,* 22 March 1898, page 7, column 3.

29 March 1899, Coates Opera House, 30th Annual Commencement

"More Doctors Graduated: The Kansas City Medical College Gives Thirty-Three the Right to Use 'M. D.,'" *Kansas City (Mo.) Daily Journal,* 30 March 1899, page 3, column 4.

"A Medical College Commencement," *Kansas City (Mo.) Star,* 29 March 1899, page 9, column 1. **(no list of graduates)**

"Another Drove of Doctors: Thirty Young Men Received Their Diplomas Last Night," *Kansas City (Mo.) Times,* 30 March 1899, page 7, column 4.

15 March 1900, Coates Opera House, 31st Annual Commencement

"Doctors Given Prizes: Commencement Exercises of the Kansas City Medical College at the Coates House," *Kansas City (Mo.) Daily Journal,* 16 March 1900, page 1, column 2. **(no list of graduates)**

"Fullfledged Doctors Now: The Kansas City Medical College Graduates Forty-Nine Students with Due Ceremony," *Kansas City (Mo.) Star,* 16 March 1900, page 4, column 2.

"Forty-Nine New Doctors Graduated: Kansas City Medical College Turns Out a Big Class—Interesting Commencement Exercises," *Kansas City (Mo.) Times,* 16 March 1900, page 6, column 6.

22 March 1901, Auditorium Theater, 32nd Annual Commencement
"Doctors Are Banqueted: Many Out of Town Guests Attend Annual Banquet of Kansas City Medical College,"
   Kansas City (Mo.) Daily Journal, 23 March 1901, page 7, column 2. **(no list of graduates)**
"Kansas City Medical College Commencement," *Kansas City (Mo.) Star,* 21 March 1901, page 5, column 2. **(no
   list of graduates)**
"Diplomas for Sixty 'Medics': The Graduation and Annual Dinner of the Kansas City Medical College," *Kansas
   City (Mo.) Star,* 23 March 1901, page 9, column 2. **(no list of graduates)**
"Degrees for New Doctors: Commencement Exercises of Kansas City Medical College Tomorrow Afternoon,"
   Kansas City (Mo.) Times, 21 March 1901, page 5, column 3. **(no list of graduates)**
"Into Field of Medicine: Forty-Three Students of the Kansas City Medical College Ready for Practical Work,"
   Kansas City (Mo.) Daily Times, 23 March 1901, page 2, column 4. **(no list of graduates)**

25 March 1902, Century Theater, 33rd Annual Commencement
"Forty-Eight New Physicians: Graduation Exercises of Two Medical Colleges to Be Held This Week," *Kansas City
   (Mo.) Daily Journal,* 25 March 1902, page 5, column 1.
"Eighteen New Doctors: Graduation Exercises of Kansas City Medical College in the Century Theater," *Kansas
   City (Mo.) Daily Journal,* 26 March 1902, page 12, column 1.
"Brief Bits of City News," *Kansas City (Mo.) Star,* 26 March 1902, page 10, column 1. **(no list of graduates)**
"It's [sic] 33d Commencement: The Graduating Exercises of the Kansas City Medical College," *Kansas City (Mo.)
   Times,* 26 March 1902, page 2, columns 4-5.

24 March 1903, Auditorium Theater, 34th Annual Commencement
"Many New Doctors: Kansas City Medical College Commencement Today," *Kansas City (Mo.) Daily Journal,* 24
   March 1903, page 5, column 3.
"More Doctors Graduated," *Kansas City (Mo.) Star,* 24 March 1903, page 2, column 1. **(no list of graduates)**
"Twenty-Four New Doctors: The Graduating Exercises of the Kansas City Medical College," *Kansas City (Mo.)
   Times,* 25 March 1903, page 2, column 3.

13 April 1904, Central High School, 35th Annual Commencement
"Twenty-Eight New Doctors: Graduated from Kansas City Medical College Last Night," *Kansas City (Mo.) Daily
   Journal,* 14 April 1904, page 3, column 5.
"Diplomas for 34 Doctors: Thirty-Third [sic] Commencement of the Kansas City Medical College To-Night,"
   Kansas City (Mo.) Times, 13 April 1904, page 4, column 2.
"Thirty-Four New Doctors: Graduating Exercises at the Kansas City Medical College Last Night," *Kansas City
   (Mo.) Times,* 14 April 1904, page 6, column 6. **(no list of graduates)**

11 April 1905, Central High School, 36th Annual Commencement
"Will Graduate a Class of 35: Commencement Exercises of the Kansas City Medical College To-Night," *Kansas
   City (Mo.) Times,* 11 April 1905, page 5, column 2. **(no list of graduates)**
"Strong's Plans for K. U.: A Great Medical School to Be Built Up, He Says," *Kansas City (Mo.) Times,* 12 April
   1905, page 2, column 3.

City Directories

1881 Kansas City, Missouri, directory, page 802:
   Kansas City Medical College. S. S. Todd, President; E. W. Schauffler, M. D., Secretary; D. R. Porter, M. D.,
   Treasurer. College building, Main, junction Delaware.
1882 Kansas City, Missouri, directory, page 619:
   Kansas City Medical College. Seventh, northwest corner Washington. E. W. Schauffler, M. D., President; F.
   M. Johnson, M. D., Secretary; D. R. Porter, Treasurer.
1883 Kansas City, Missouri, directory, page 525:
   Kansas City Medical College. Seventh, northwest corner Washington. E. W. Schauffler, M. D., President; F.
   M. Johnson, M. D., Secretary; D. R. Porter, Treasurer.

Kansas City Medical College (continued)

1884 Kansas City, Missouri, directory, page 674:
Kansas City Medical College. Seventh, northwest corner Washington. E. W. Schauffler, M. D., President; F. M. Johnson, M. D., Secretary; D. R. Porter, Treasurer.

1885 Kansas City, Missouri, directory, age 710:
Kansas City Medical College, Seventh, northwest corner Washington.

1886 Kansas City, Missouri, directory, page 993:
Kansas City Medical College—Seventh, northwest corner Washington.

1887 Kansas City, Missouri, directory, page 821:
Kansas City Medical College, 628 Washington

1888 Kansas City, Missouri, directory, page 383:
Kansas City Medical College, 628 Washington, E. W. Schauffler, M. D. pres. Jacob Block, M. D. sec. D. R. Porter, M. D. treas

1889 Kansas City, Missouri, directory, page 370:
Kansas City Medical College, 628 Washington E. W. Schauffler M. D. pres D. R. Porter M. D. treas

1890 Kansas City, Missouri, directory, page 375:
Kansas City Medical College, 628 Washington E. W. Schauffler pres D. R. Porter sec and treas

1891 Kansas City, Missouri, directory, page 355:
Kansas City Medical College, 628 Washington E. W. Schauffler pres Joseph Sharp sec

1892 Kansas City, Missouri, directory, page 327:
Kansas City Medical College, 628 Washington J. D. Griffith pres; Joseph Sharp sec

1893 Kansas City, Missouri, directory, page 745:
Kansas City Medical College, 628 Wash'n. J. D. Griffith, pres; Jos. Sharp, sec.

1894 Kansas City, Missouri, directory, page 754:
Kansas City Medical College, 628 Wash'n, E. W. Schauffler pres; Jos. Sharp, sec.

1895 Kansas City, Missouri, directory, page 858:
Kansas City Medical College, 628 Wash'n, E. W. Schauffler pres; Jos. Sharp, sec.

1896 Kansas City, Missouri, directory, page 900:
Kansas City Medical College, 628 Wash'n, J. D. Griffith, Dean; E. W. Schauffler Pres; F. E. Murphy, Sec.

1897 Kansas City, Missouri, directory, page 887:
Kansas City Medical College, 628 Wash'n, J. D. Griffith, Dean; E. W. Schauffler Pres; F. E. Murphy, Sec.

1898 Kansas City, Missouri, directory, page 967:
Kansas City Medical College, 628 Wash'n. J. D. Griffith, Dean; E. W. Schauffler, Pres; F. E. Murphy, Sec.

1899 Kansas City, Missouri, directory, page 1084:
Kansas City Medical College, 628 Wash'n. J. D. Griffith, Dean; E. W. Schauffler, Pres; F. E. Murphy, Sec.

1900 Kansas City, Missouri, directory, page 1293:
Kansas City Medical College, 628 Wash'n. A. L. Fulton, Dean; E. W. Schauffler, Pres; F. E. Murphy, Sec.

1901 Kansas City, Missouri, directory, page 582:
Kansas City Medical College 628 Washn, Dr E W Schauffler pres, Dr J H VanEman v-pres, Dr W C Tyree sec, Dr D R Porter treas, Dr A L Fulton dean

1902 Kansas City, Missouri, directory, page 628:
Kansas City Medical College 628 Washn, Dr R T Sloan dean, Dr Robt McE Schauffler sec of faculty

1903 Kansas City, Missouri, directory, page 642:
Kansas City Medical College 628 Washn Dr R T Sloan dean, Dr Robt McE Schauffler sec of faculty

1904 Kansas City, Missouri, directory, page 650:
Kansas City Medical College 628 Washn, Dr R T Sloan dean, Dr Robt McE Schauffler sec of faculty

1905 Kansas City, Missouri, directory, page 607:
Kansas City Medical College 628 Washn Dr E W Schauffler pres Dr T J Beattie sec Dr D R Porter treas

Medical Department of the University of Kansas City (1881-1889)

Medical Department of the University of Kansas City was established in 1881 and its first graduating class was in 1882. In 1890 its name was changed to University Medical College (1890-1913).

Surname	Given Names	City	State	Remarks
1882				
Ambrose	J. A.		KS	
Auerbach	Louis	Berlin	Prussia	
Bigger	D. P.	Kansas City	MO	Honorary Degree
Bills	A. R.		CO	
Burke	C. L.			
Clayton	Z. C.		KS	
Cookerly	C. E.	Kansas City	MO	
Malone	S. L.		KS	
Morse	Silas E.		IA	Valedictorian
Still	J. J.		KS	
Williamson	G. W.		KS	
1883				
Caughill	Frank A.	Chamois	MO	Prize
Friedenberg	Eugene L.	Kansas City	MO	
Gossett	John W.	Paola	KS	
Logan	James E.	Kansas City	MO	Prize
Peters	Alexander B.	Salem	KS	
Schmitz	Albert F.	Sedalia	MO	Prize
Scholl	Grayson B.	Girard	KS	
Snell	Dupuy	Clay County	MO	Prize
1884				
Cathcart	Charles P./T.	Kansas City	MO	
Chase	Thomas	Rosedale / Shawneetown	KS	
Coonce	George W.	Boone County	MO	
Craig	William E.	Kansas City	MO	
Ewin	Charles E.	Independence	MO	Prize
Harkins	Hugh C.	Saint Louis	MO	Valedictorian; 2 Prizes
Johnston/Johnson	Samuel A./R.	Saint Charles	MO	
Kernodle	Oliver P.	Sedalia	MO	
Magill	Isaac H.		KS	
Mayginnes	M./N. W.	Mound Valley	KS	Prize
Robinson	John S.	Calhoun	MO	
Tidmore	James A.	White Church	KS	
Wohlfahrth/Wolfordt	Lewis A.	Rosedale	KS	
Wood	Harry B./D.	Kansas City	MO	

Surname	Given Names	City	State	Remarks
1885				
Brooks	S. H.			
Dennis	E. J.			Prize
Dunning	Franklin L.			
Findlay	C. H.			Valdictorian
Hunt	A. L.			
Jackson	W.			
Lewis	W. W.			
Moses	J. E.			
Rogers	S. L.			
Secrost	J. F.			
Sheeler	D. W.			
Short	John L.			
Thornton	W. N.			
Wear	R. C.			
Wesselowski	Julius			Prize
Wilkes	William O.	Waco	TX	2 Prizes
1886				
Addington	C. H.		KS	
Armstrong	T. R.		IA	Prize (Instruments)
Bigger	T. H.	Brainerd	MN	
Brown	George H.	Chanute	KS	
Bryant	John W.	Clay County	MO	Prize ($25)
Carhart	E. L.	Wilson	KS	Prize
Frazer	William T.		WA Territory	
Green	R. L.	Kansas City	MO	Prize (Book)
Hill	John R.	Fayette	AR	
Horn	M. L.	Fairfield	IA	Valedictorian
Meisner	W. H.	Mulberry Grove	KS	
Mentzer	O. F.		Sweden	
Myers	O. P.	Joplin	MO	
Smith	H. G.		KS	
Smith	L. J.	Denver	CO	
Spencer	T. C.		TX	
Van Wagner	E. J.	Kansas City	MO	
1887				
Anderson	Victor			
Lilly	G. W.			
Merriman	Clay S.			Valedictorian
Milner	John Orr			
Thornton	J. D.			
Waring	B. B.			

Medical Department of the University of Kansas City (continued)

Surname	Given Names	City	State	Remarks
1888				
Baum	Fritz			
Compton	Fred			
Jeffries	C. A./O.			4 Prizes
Jones	Horatio S.			Prize
Kelley	Andrew			
Mooney	J. H./W.			
Wilkins	W. F. / F. J.			
Young	S. V.			2 Prizes
1889				
Bagley	B. H.			
Brewer	J. F.			Prize
Falconer	A.			
Hamilton	C. C.			Prize
Harrington	J. L.			2 Prizes
Kiefer	J. G.			
McDonald	P. L.			Prize
Middlebrook	Edmond			
Mindor	W. E.			Prize
Payne	E. B.			Prize
Rairdon	C. W.			
Rice	J. T.			Prize
Russell	J. J.			
Steenborg	W. B.			Prize
Wright	C.			

Newspapers

02 March 1882, First Baptist Church, 1st Annual Commencement
"The First: Commencement Exercises of the University of Kansas City, in the Medical Department," *Kansas City (Mo.) Daily Journal,* 03 March 1882, page 4, column2 5-6, page 5, columns 1-2.
"Dawning Doctors: Commencement Exercises of the Medical Department of the University of Kansas City," *Kansas City (Mo.) Star,* 03 March 1882, page 1, column 4.
"More M. D.'s,: The University of Kansas City Turns Out Ten graduates To-Night," *Kansas City (Mo.) Times,* 02 March 1882, page 8, column 2.
"Full Fledged Doctors: Commencement Exercises at the University of Kansas City," *Kansas City (Mo.) Times,* 03 March 1882, page 8, columns 1-4, page 5, column 4.

13 March 1883, Walnut Street Methodist Episcopal Church (South), 2nd Annual Commencement
"University of Kansas City," *Kansas City (Mo.) Daily Journal,* 14 March 1883, page 3, column 1.
"Fresh Fledged Physicians: Another Galaxy of Them Turned Loose Last Night," *Kansas City (Mo.) Star,* 14 March 1883, page 1, column 2.
"Commencement Exercises," *Kansas City (Mo.) Times,* 14 March 1883, page 5, column 1.

13 March 1884, Walnut Street Methodist Episcopal Church (South), 3rd Annual Commencement
"University Commencement," *Kansas City (Mo.) Daily Journal,* 14 March 1884, page 3, column 1.
"Medical Matters," *Kansas City (Mo.) Star,* 14 March 1884, page 1, column 4. **(no list of graduates)**
"Commencement Exercises," *Kansas City (Mo.) Times,* 10 Mar 1884, page 8, column 5.

"Doctors' Degrees Conferred: Interesting and Successful Commencement Exercises Last Evening—A Brilliant Banquet," *Kansas City (Mo.) Times,* 14 March 1884, page 5, column 1.

11 March 1885, Walnut Street Methodist Episcopal Church (South), 4th Annual Commencement
"Commencement Exercises," *Kansas City (Mo.) Daily Journal,* 12 March 1885, page 3, columns 2-4. **(no list of graduates)**
"Commencement Exercises," *Kansas City (Mo.) Star,* 12 March 1885, page 2, column 4. **(no list of graduates)**
"Doctors' Diplomas," Graduating Exercises of the Medical Department of the University of Kansas City," *Kansas City (Mo.) Times,* 12 March 1885, page 8, column 2.

11 March 1886, Music Hall, 5th Annual Commencement
"A Batch of M. D.'s," *Kansas City (Mo.) Daily Journal,* 12 March 1886, page 3, column 2.
"Graduating Exercises: Seventeen Medical Doctors Turned Loose—Address by Dr. Laws—Prizes Awarded," *Kansas City (Mo.) Star,* 12 March 1886, page 2, column 3.
"Making M. D.'s: Seventeen Turned Out by the University of Kansas City Last Night," *Kansas City (Mo.) Times,* 12 March 1886, page 5, column 1.

17 March 1887, Music Hall, 6th Annual Commencement
"Medical Commencement,' *Kansas City (Mo.) Daily Journal,* 18 March 1887, page 3, columns 4-5.
"City News Condensed," *Kansas City (Mo.) Star,* 18 March 1887, page 1, column 4.
"Six New Doctors: The Graduating Exercises of the University Medical Class—Interesting Addresses Made," *Kansas City (Mo.) Times,* 18 March 1887, page 2, column 5.

15 March 1888, Music Hall, 7th Annual Commencement
"Graduates in Medicine: The Seventh Annual Commencement of the Medical Department of the University of Kansas City," *Kansas City (Mo.) Daily Journal,* 16 March 1888, page 3, column 2.
""Commencement Exercises: Degrees Conferred upon Graduates of Two Medical Colleges," *Kansas City (Mo.) Times,* 16 March 1888, page 8, column 2.

14 March 1889, Music Hall, 8th or 9th Annual Commencement
"Fifteen New Doctors of Medicine," *Kansas City (Mo.) Star,* 15 March 1889, page 1, column 1.
"Fifteen More Doctors: Graduating Exercises of the Medical Department of University of Kansas City," *Kansas City (Mo.) Times,* 15 March 1889, page 5, column 2.

City Directories

1880 Kansas City, Missouri, directory   —
1881 Kansas City, Missouri, directory   —
1882 Kansas City, Missouri, directory, page 619:
    University of Kansas City. Twelfth, s. e. cor. McGee. Board of Regents: Nathan Scarrett [sic.], D. D. LL. D., President; John R. Snell, M. D., Vice-President; Flavel B. Tiffany, M. D., Secretary; Edward L. Martin, Treasurer; Hon. Robert E. Cowan, Thomas B. Bullene, J. W. Jackson, M.D. Officers of the Medical Department.: Henry F. Hereford, M. D., President; John R. Snell, M. D., Dean; Geo. M. Bergen, M. D., Secretary; Gonzalo E. Buxton, M. D., Treasurer.
1883 Kansas City, Missouri, directory, page 525:
    University of Kansas City. Twelfth, southeast corner McGee. Officers of the Medical Department. Henry F. Hereford, M. D., President; John R. Snell, M. D., Dean; George H. Chapman, M. D., Secretary; C. W. Adams, M. D., Treasurer.
1884 Kansas City, Missouri, directory, page 674:
    University of Kansas City. Twelfth, southeast cor McGee. Officers of the Medical Department. Henry F. Hereford, M. D., President; John R. Snell, M. D., Dean; J. W. Elston, M. D., Secretary; C. W. Adams, M. D., Treasurer.

1885 Kansas City, Missouri, directory, page 710:

University of Kansas City. Twelfth, southeast cor. McGee. Officers of the Medical Department. Henry F. Hereford, M. D., President; John R. Snell, M. D., Dean; J. W. Elston, M. D., Secretary; C. W. Adams, M. D., Treasurer.

1886 Kansas City, Missouri, directory, page 993:

University of Kansas City. Twelfth, southeast corner McGee, J. W. Jackson, President; J. E. Logan, Secretary; G. W. Davis, Treasurer; J. R. Snell, Dean.

1887 Kansas City, Missouri, directory, page 821:

University of Kansas City, Medical Department, J. W. Jackson, M. D., president; James E. Logan, M. D., secretary, 12th, south-east corner McGee

1888 Kansas City, Missouri, directory, page 897:

University of Kansas City (Medical Department), 911 east 10th. J. W. Jackson, president; J. R. Snell, dean; S. E. Lanphear [sic], secretary.

1889 Kansas City, Missouri, directory, page 880:

University of Kansas City (Medical department), 911 east 10th. J. W. Jackson, Pres.; J. P. Jackson, Dean; S. E. Lanphear [sic], Sec.

Medico-Chirurgical College
(1898-1905)

Medico-Chirurgical College, established in 1898, was formerly Kansas City [KS] College of Medicine and Surgery (1896-1898). Its first graduating class was in 1898. In 1905 this school merged with Kansas City Medical College (1880-1905) and College of Physicians and Surgeons of the Kansas City [KS] University (1894-1905), forming School of Medicine of the University of Kansas (1905-).

Surname	Given Names	City	State	Remarks
1898				
Krugg	A. A.			
1899				
Bleil	Albert Willis			
Fortner	Charles Hughes/Hugh			Prize (Instruments)
Harris	Edgar Sander			Prize ($10)
Mount	James Rudolph			Prize (Books)
Rogers	Alfred Hezekiah (AM)			Prize (Instruments)
Smith	John Ellsworth			
1900				
Black	Roy Leslie			
Bradford	George Washington			
Bredehoft	Julius Curt			
Burrows	Agin			
Corn	John Asa			
Crabtree	John Smith			
Gastwiler	John Schooling			
Jenkins	William Henry			
Lee	Richard Henry			
Major	Clive			
Moberly	Robert Lindsay			
Pate	Jacob Edmond			
Pelt	Levi Alexander			
Reed	David William			
Ross	Harry Reath			
Rowell	Hiram Jennings			
Thompson	George Byron			
Vineyard	Samuel Polk			
Westlake	Oliver James			
Williams	Robert Alvin			

Surname	**Given Names**	**City**	**State**	**Remarks**

1901

Bickers	J. B.			
Booth	L. R.			
Brown	C. H.			
Cleverdon	L. A.			
DeTar	Monroe			
Duncan	A. L.			
Fisher	C. A.			
Gilliland	V. E.			
Johnson	F./J. G.			
Parker	F. R.			
Reed/Reid	J. T.			
Richards	J. G./J.			
Suwalsky	Albert L.			
Talman/Tatman	M./W. H.			

1902

Berry	George Washington			
Bickel	Charles			
Candler	Fred Day			
Chadwick	Ira Bradford			
Coffin	Benjamin Franklin			
Cornell	Harry Leslie (AM)			
Davis	Jefferson Allen			
Howell	David William			
McManis	James Edwin			
McMullin	Verbena			
Pinkston	James Anderson			
Pipkin	George Phillip (AB)			
Porter	William Avin (DVS)			
Rhoads	Mark Herbert (BS)			
Voegelin	Samuel			

1903

Barber	Andrew Hamilton			
Berry	George Washington			
Blain	Fred Otto			
Brownfield	Robert Roy			
Grace	John Franklin			
Grace	Thomas Andrew			
Hammontree	Daniel Edward (Hammondtree)			
Hartford	Isaac James (BS)			
Howard	Charles			
Kyle	Thomas Rufus			
LaRue	Harper Miles			
Lieurance	Edward			
Morrow	Earl Joseph			

Surname	**Given Names**	**City**	**State**	**Remarks**

1903 Continues

Newton	Littleton Alexander			
Osell	Arvin/Arvid Emanuel (AB)			
Porter	William Avin (DVS)			
Powell	James Thomas (BS)			
Ragan	Romulus Claiborne			
Smith	J. Clyde			
Smith	Joseph Green			
Swaney	William Daniel			

1904

Case	James H.			
Dever	Harvey A.			
Heaath	J. F.			
Isley	Charles F.			
Kane	James H.			
Kirkham	Arch			
Klock	Ross F.			
LaRue	Harper M.			
Matthews	John H.			
Moore	Watson A.			
Nickson	Charles E.			
Ralston	James H.			
Rentfro	Emmet W.			
Salyer	C. E.			
Shepard	John W.			
Smith	B. P.			
Van de Sand	W. B.			
Webber	G. E.			
Wood	Delbert L.			

Newspapers

31 March 1899, Academy of Music, 2nd Annual Commencement

"Kansas City Homeopathic College," *Kansas City (Mo.) Daily Journal,* 16 March 1899, page 7, column 3.

"Six Got Diplomas: Annual Commencement Exercises of the Medico-Chirurgical College Last Night," *Kansas City (Mo.) Daily Journal,* 01 April 1899, page 7, column 1.

"To Graduate Eight Doctors: The Commencement Exercises of the Medico-Chirurgical College To-Night," *Kansas City (Mo.) Star,* 31 March 1899, page 10, column 2.

"Commencement Is Held: Students of the Medico-Chirurgical College Receive Diplomas," *Kansas City (Mo.) Times,* 01 April 1899, page 4, column 7.

13 March 1900, Academy of Music, 3rd Annual Commencement

"Twenty New Doctors: The Medico-Chirurgical College to Confer Degrees Tuesday Evening," *Kansas City (Mo.) Star,* 11 March 1900, page 4, column 4.

20 March 1901, Academy of Music, 4th Annual Commencement
"Fourteen Graduates: Degree of 'M. D.' Conferred by Medico-Chirurgical College—Banquet at the Midland,"
   Kansas City (Mo.) Daily Journal, 21 March 1901, page 10, column 4.
"Diplomas for Young Doctors: A Class of Fourteen Was Graduated from the Medico-Chirurgical College," *Kansas
   City (Mo.) Star,* 21 March 1901, page 4, column 1.

20 March 1902, Academy of Music, 5th Annual Commencement
"Are Given Their Diplomas: The Commencement Exercises of the Medico-Chirurgical College Last Night," *Kansas
   City (Mo.) Daily Journal,* 21 March 1902, page 7, column 2.
"Medico-Chi Commencement: Fifteen in This Year's Graduating Class of College," *Kansas City (Mo.) Star,* 16
   March 1902, page 11, column 4.
"The 'Medico-Chi' Commencement," *Kansas City (Mo.) Star,* 21 March 1902, page 4, column 3.
"Fifteen Doctors Graduated: Commencement Exercises of the Medi[c]o Chirrugical College," *Kansas City (Mo.)
   Times,* 21 March 1902, page 2, column 2.

19 March 1903, Academy of Music, 6[th] Annual Commencement
"To Turn Out Doctors: Two Medical Schools to Hold Graduations This Month," *Kansas City (Mo.) Daily Journal,*
   18 March 1903, page 5, column 2.
"Twenty New Doctors: Graduating Exercises of the Medico-Chirurgical College Last Night," *Kansas City (Mo.)
   Times,* 20 March 1903, page 6, column 6.

02 April 1904, [unknown venue], 7th Annual Commencement
"Diplomas for Doctors: A Class of Nineteen Graduated by Medico-Chirurgical College," *Kansas City (Mo.) Star,* 03
   April 1904, page 9, column 2.

12 April 1905, Central High School, 8th Annual Commencement
"Sixteen More Doctors Graduated," *Kansas City (Mo.) Times,* 13 April 1905, page 2, column 2. **(no list of
   graduates)**
"To Graduate Tonight: Class from Medico-Chirurgical College Will Receive Diplomas and Banquet," *Kansas City
   (Mo.) World,* 12 April 1905, page 1, column 2. **(no list of graduates)**

City Directories

1899 Kansas City, Missouri, directory, page 1084:
   Medico-Chirurgical College, 409 Cherry. Dr. G. O. Coffin, Dean; Dr. J. L. Harrington, Sec.
1900 Kansas City, Missouri, directory, page 1298:
   Medico-Chirurgical College, 409 Cherry. Dr. G. O. Coffin, Dean; Dr. J. L. Harrington, Sec.
1901 Kansas City, Missouri, directory, page 736:
   Medico-Chirurgical College 409-411 Cherry Dr G O Coffin dean, Dr J L Harrington sec
1902 Kansas City, Missouri, directory, page 797:
   Medico-Chirurgical College 914-918 Inde av Dr C L Hall pres, Dr B L Eastman v-pres, Dr J L Harrington sec,
   Dr W F Kuhn treas, Dr G O Coffin dean
1903 Kansas City, Missouri, directory, page 801:
   Medico-Chirurgical College 914-918 Inde av Dr C L Hall pres, Dr B L Eastman v-pres, Dr J L Harrington sec,
   Dr B E Fryer treas, Dr G O Coffin dean
1904 Kansas City, Missouri, directory, page 322:
   Medico-Chirurgical College 914-918 Inde av Dr G O Coffin –pres Dr B E Fryer v-pres Dr J L Harrington sec
   Dr L G Taylor treas Dr C Lester Hall dean
1905 Kansas City, Missouri, directory, page 770:
   Medico-Chirurgical College 914-918 Inde av Dr G O Coffin pres Dr B E Fryer vpres Dr J L Harrington sec Dr
   L G Taylor treas Dr C L Hall dean

National School and Infirmary of Osteopathy (1897-ca. 1901)

National School and Infirmary of Osteopathy was founded in 1897. No record of graduating classes has been found. The Osteopathic College in Kirksville sued this school, accusing it of selling diplomas to persons who had not taken classes. This college last appears in directories of Kansas City, Missouri, in 1901.

Newspapers

[unknown date] 1898, [unknown venue], Annual Commencement

[unknown date] 1899, [unknown venue], Annual Commencement

[unknown date] 1900, [unknown venue], Annual Commencement

[unknown date] 1901, [unknown venue], Annual Commencement

[unknown date] 1902, [unknown venue], Annual Commencement

[unknown date] 1903, [unknown venue], Annual Commencement

[unknown date] 1904, [unknown venue], Annual Commencement

[unknown date] 1905, [unknown venue], Annual Commencement

City Directories

1895 Kansas City, Missouri, directory   —
1896 Kansas City, Missouri, directory   —
1897 Kansas City, Missouri, directory, page 502:
    NATIONAL SCHOOL AND INFIRMARY OF OSTEOPATHY, 415 to 418 K & P bldg, Dr W A Cormack
    pres; Helen M Barberry v-pres; E D Barber treas. See Physicians
1898 Kansas City, Missouri, directory, page 551:
    NATIONAL SCHOOL AND INFIRMARY OF OSTEOPATHY, 415 to 428 K & P bldg tel 2814, E D Barber
    pres and treas; Helen M Barber v-pres; A L Barber sec
1899 Kansas City, Missouri, directory, page 1084:
    National School & Infirmary of Osteopathy, 407 to 412 Hall bldg. [Walnut nw cor 9th] L. W. Welsh Dean.
1900 Kansas City, Missouri, directory, page 1298:
    National School & Infirmary of Osteopathy, 407 to 412 Hall bldg. [Walnut nw cor 9th] L. W. Welsh, Dean.
1901 Kansas City, Missouri, directory, page 795:
    NATIONAL SCHOOL & INFIRMARY OF OSTEOPATHY, 407 to 412 Hall bldg, [Walnut nw cor 9th] tel
    2814 Dr E D Barber pres, Helen M Barber v-pres, A L Barber sec, L W Welsh dean See initial letter "O" [ad]
1902 Kansas City, Missouri, directory   —
1903 Kansas City, Missouri, directory   —

University Medical College
(1890-1913)

University Medical College, established in 1890, was formerly Medical Department of the University of Kansas City (1881-1889). Its first graduating class was in 1890. In 1913 this school was disbanded.

Surname	Given Names	City	State	Remarks
1890				
Atkins	Calvin			3 Prizes
Barney	Reuben			2 Prizes
Bradley	M. E.			
Clarke	William J.			
Corwin	L. A.			
Coulson	J. R.			
Dalgliesh	George D.			
Elliott	Ira T.			
Grover	Charles M.			2 Prizes
Iles	W. A.			
Johnson	W. M.			
Salisbury	Harry T.			Prize
Sevier	Robert E.			
Thornton	Thomas E.			
Wilson	B. F.			
1891				
Benson	Thomas Clarkson	Kansas City	KS	
Bowman	Alfred R.	La Due	MO	
Brennan	Thomas Francis	Kansas City	MO	
Cox	Miley E.	Kansas City	MO	
Elmore	John Lee	Kansas City	MO	
Ewin	William Henry	Independence	MO	
Fraker	George W., Jr.	Excelsior Springs	MO	
Green	Luther D.	Kansas City	MO	
Griswold	Edward Harry	New Haven	MO	
Jackson	Jabez North	Kansas City	MO	Prize (Instruments)
James	Charles Stephen	Centerville	IA	
Jerowitz	Hermann David	Kansas City	MO	Prize ($100)
Jones	Elijah	McLouth	KS	
Kackley	Lord Byron	Chetopa	KS	
Lincoln	Ben S.	Kearney	MO	
McDonald	Chett	Kansas City	MO	
Medaris	James Henderson	Harper	KS	
Meradith	Charles S.	Montezuma	KS	
Minor	James Carl	Chillicothe	MO	
Monks	Frederick Coston	Kittaning	PA	
Moore	Osborne Lee	Spring Garden	MO	
Parker	Charles Weakley	Kansas City	MO	
Ravenscraft	Noah Davod	Smithville	MO	

Surname	Given Names	City	State	Remarks
1891 Continues				
Van Schoiack	Frank H.	Ottawa	KS	
Waful	Charles C.	Lathrop	MO	
Wilson	Albert Miller	Kansas City	KS	
Wilson	Charles F.	Booneville	TX	
Wood	Leroy Mayoon	White Church	KS	
Wood	Watson Fuller	Cumberland County	VA	
Wooton	Marion Washington	Purdy	MO	
1892				
Alexander	W. B.			
Bacon	G. H.			
Brewer	E. E.			
Brooks	T.			
Brown	J. W.			Prize
Burke	W. C.			Prize
Dix	Thomas A.			
Doyle	T.			
Edwards	A. G.			
Ennis	J. M.			
Forest	James D.			
Fulton	F. H.			
Goben	Horace G.			
Greenlee	Aubrey R.			
Harms	J. H.			
Harrison	E. Lee			
Henry	Buford M.			
Jennings	Williston T.			
Lowrey	W. J.			
Markham	Robert M.			
Martin	C. P.			
McCarty	George D.			
McFarland	A. F.			
Moffett	C. B.			
Moore	D. J.			
Murphy	Archibald			
Richards	George W.			
Roh	Carl F.			
Schaefer	E. H.			
Shaw	B. F.			
Stephens	Charles E.			
Strieby	U. G.			
Waite	W. F.			
Willard	Henry S.			
Wingo	Nova W.			
Woods	I. M.			
Woods	R. A.			

Surname	Given Names	City	State	Remarks
1893				
Alexander	William B.			
Bly	Theron Harrison			
Darby	Robert Ezra			
Dold	William Addison			
Dowell	Robert Lee			
Egelston/Eggelston	John Chester			
Gaines	John Joseph			
Hayden	B. S. "Doc" John			
Haynes	John Roger			Prize ($100)
Jones	Edgar H.			
Maxson	John Child (PhG)			
Settle	James Albert			
Shepherd	Homer E.			
Tihan/Tihen	Herman B.			
Waite	William Finley			
Welch	Thomas Edgar (AB)			Prize
White	William L.			
Wunnicke	August C.			
1894				
Adamson	L. P.			
Ames	E. W.			Prize ($100)
Chace	E. P.			
Draper	T. J.			
Gossett	E. B.			
Hawthorne	Edward W. (AG)			
Hollenbeck	A. G.			
Jaquith	J. H.			
Ludwick	Arthur L.			
McConnell	W. C.			
Myers	James T.			
Neff	Robert L.			Prize (Instruments)
Parker	Ivan B.			
Schneider	Jacob A.			
Scott	A. B.			
Springsteen	Benjamin F.			
Turner	Frank S.			
Ussher	B. B. (Bishop)			
Webber	P. O.			
1895				
Albright	Henry C.			
Armstrong	Elwood			
Bennefeld	Alfred			
Bradley	Charles Edward			
Brierly	Henry A.			

Surname	Given Names	City	State	Remarks
1895 Continues				
Cain	Milton			
Emery	Frank W.			
Farrer	George William			
Gardner	Wesley J.			
Gerard	Ed N., Jr.			
Greaves	Eli A.			
Greaves	Joseph			
Green	David E.			
Harrison	Alvin F.			Prize ($100)
Hyde	Bennet Clark			
Jeans	J. W.			
Kready	Jacob H.			
Lieberman	B. Albert			
Lloyd	H. Charles			
Mather	Harry F.			
McMurtry	Thomas A.			
Mitchell	A. R.			
Oglesby	James V.			
O'Neil	F. E			
Porter	Emerson S.			
Rennick	Charles W.			
Riley	Frank L.			
Ritchey	William W.			
Simpson	Arthur J.			
Smythe	Charles H.			
Southern	John N.			
Sulzbacher	Bruno L.			Prize (Instruments)
Thomas	Arthur W.			
Todd	Elhanan H.			
Woods	Samuel H.			
1896				
Albritain	J. W.			
Boarman	J. A.			
Brown	R. J.			
Cantwell	B. T.			
Chapman	O. M.			
Clopper	D. E.			
Cole	T. C.			
Davis	G. W.			
Davis	O. P.			
Dillenbeck	F. E.			
Donaldson	J. E.			
Downing	J. L.			
Drane	J. E.			
Field	W. S.			
Findley	M. C.			

Surname	Given Names	City	State	Remarks
1896 Continues				
Galloway	G. R.			
Giles	Harry L.	Shelbina	MO	Prize (Instruments)
Girdner	W. M.			
Glynn	G. C.			
Goodman	G.			
Gregg	A. C.			
Hall	D. W.			
Halstead	J. W.			
Hinton	W. H.	Ottawa	KS	Prize ($100)
Hollis	L. T.			
Hultner	A.			
Hymer	J. E.			
Kunze	H.			
Landon	S. S.			
Lichtenberg	J. S.			
Lothian	W.			
Lutz	T. E.			
Mahaffy	G. C.			
McMillan	D. J. (DDS)			
Moore	G. W. H.			
Newell	T. G.			
Nickell	C. A.			
Parker	W. W.			
Platter	A. E.			
Plunkett	D. J.			
Proud	W. C.			
Reeds	I. M.			
Ryburn	R. H.			
Scott	J. S.			
Steadman	L. S.			
Stephan	J. J.			
Stocks	C. L.			
Turner	F. W. R.			
Ussher	C. D.			
Wheeler	H. R.			
Williams	G.			
Wilson	L. S.			
1897				
Agin	Burroughs			
Andersson	H. C.			
Ashley	G. L. R.			
Ballaine	C. W.			
Bernhardt	W. H.			
Berry	George F.			
Boling	R. L.			

Surname	Given Names	City	State	Remarks
1897 Continues				
Brown	T. O.			
Bryan	J. R.			
Bushong	L. Bittle			
Carpenter	A. L.			
Clinton	F. S. (PhG)			
Coffey	A. McD.			
Cook	F. L.			
Cumpton	V. J.			
Davenport	R. G.			
Day	Fred K.			
Devin	J. F.			
Dieuis	R. O.			
Donaven	E. A. (BS)			
Edwards	W. R. J.			
Ellis	Frank B.			
Emes	Charles A.			
Everhardy	J. L. (AM)			
Fisher	F. B. (BS)	Springfield	IL	Prize (Instruments)
Frizell	L. N. (PhG)			
Gage	G. R. (PhG)			
Greason	W. B. (AB)			
Greer	T. S.			
Gross	J. F.			
Harrison	W. H.			
Henderson	A. J.			
Hendricks	H. L.			
Hepler	A. H.			
Jackson	C. A. (PhG)			
James	W. A. (AB)			
Johnson	W. E.			
Joiner	G. W.			
King	W. E. (PhD)			
Lapp	John G.			
Lehew	John L.			
Lemon	James G.			
Leverich	L.			
Lingenfelter	G. P.			
Loughridge	S.			
Maupin	R. E.			
Mayberry	E. A.			
McAllister	N. E.			
McHenry	Dolph D.			
Meador	C. A.			
Montgomery	W. E.			
Morrison	A. (PhG)			
Morton	George			

Surname	Given Names	City	State	Remarks
1897 Continues				
Myers	Mark C.			
Neff	Frank C.			
Norberg	G. B. (PhD)			
Norman	Edward J.			
O'Donnell	Fred W.			
Parker	O. T. (PhG)			
Phillips	Solomon			
Phy	William T.	Union City	OR	Prize ($100)
Rice	William			
Richmond	Thomas			
Roberts	W. W.			
Rowell	F. D. (DVS)			
Scott	J. N. (PhG)			
Seright	J. H.			
Shawhan	R. C.			
Shouse	Charles			
Shoyer	Mayer			
Standley	E. D. (MS)			
Swatlander	J. C.			
Tenny	Edwin R.			
Thomas	M. U.			
Thomas	W. M.			
Thompson	C. E.			
Thompson	S. G.			
Tureman	H. G.			
Wanamaker	A. E.			
Wattles	J. H. (DVS)			
Woodson	W. H., Jr.			
Wright	Uriel S.			
Zimmerman	A. C.			
1898				
Barger	J. N.			
Berger	Fred			
Boone	J. W. C.			
Bryson	E. H.			
Cairnes	James			
Christianson	M.			
Cooper	C. L.			
Durrant	Ira E.			
Farnsworth	A. D.			
Farrar	W. A.			
Gerhart	A. P.			
Goelitz	H. W.			Prize (Instruments)
Hall	O. B.			
Henderson	L. E.			

Surname	Given Names	City	State	Remarks
1898 Continues				
Hoagland	W. L.			
Humphreys	J. E.			
Lahmer	I. B.			
Lane	H. H.			
Lane	Wallace C.			
Lee	H. C.			
Lemmon	J. G.			
Light	R. A.			
Long	L. L.			
Lowdermilk	R. C.			Prize (Instruments)
Marquis	T. B.			
McArthur	Arthur W.			
McIlwain	W.			
Middleton	James			
Miller	S. J.			
Moore	Samuel			
Morphis	L. B.			
Moulder	T. V.			
Murtaugh	E. G.			
Myers	S. S.			
Mynatt	A. J.			
Newhouse	Stanley			
Parker	T. F.			
Peak	Frank			
Pierce	J. L.			
Pleher	F. W.			
Saunders	F. L.			Prize ($100)
Schmitt	G. L.			
Searl	O. R.			
Shoener	Joseph			
Sloan	E. P.			
Smith	W. C.			
Snook	T. A.			
Stafford	G. A.			
Sutton	F. R.			
Sweeney	J. L.			
Tanner	W. C.			
Taylor	J. M.			
Tees	F. D.			
Temple	I. U.			
Thomson	A.			
Thomson	A. M.			
Toomey	W. H.			
Vickers	C. P.			
Warner	T. W.			
Weyant	Z. H.			

Surname	Given Names	City	State	Remarks
1898 Continues				
Willis	H. T.			
Wooding	W. W.			
Woods	E. A.			
Wright	G. D.			
Wysong	W. L.			
Yost	J. E.			
1899				
Allen	Edward T.			Prize (Instruments)
Ayre	P. S.			
Barnes	H. M.			
Barney	H. N.			
Bowers	E. T.			
Breckenridge	J. C.			
Brubacher	J.			
Chittenden	H. W.			
Cook	C. F. N.			
Cooper	H. B.			
Cutherson	W. K.			
Cyrene	C. E.			
Davis	W. L.			
Dwight	M. K.			
Eldridge	J. S.			
Gale	R. G.			
Garrett	H. W.			
Gerard	G. R.			
Gould	E. G.			
Hampton	T. J.			Prize (Instruments)
Henly/Henley/Hendy	W. R.			
Hewett	J. E.			
Higdon	E. T.			
Hill	C. B.			
Hockaday	C. V.			
Jones	H. F.			
Kinsey	J. F.			
Loughridge	V. J.			
Ludlum	Elmer			
Lusk	B. E.			
Moore	R. W.			
Murray	D. S.			
Pendleton	E. F.			
Randall	T. J.			
Ray	Richard			
Reed	E./F. P.			
Rice	F. D.			
Rush	J. E.			

Surname	Given Names	City	State	Remarks
1899 Continues				
Shouse	Edward			
Slater	E./H. F.			
Sulzbacher	Carl I.			
Thompson	G. C.			
Tilton	A. L.			Prize ($100)
Tralle	G. M.			
Wall	E. J.			
Walthal	J. D.			
Watson	F. L.			
Weir	E. F.			
Wells	S. N.			
Williams	E. D.			
Williams	W. R.			
Williamson	C. N.			
Wood	W. R.			
1900				
Aleshire	J. Lenne			
Anderson	Arthur Lynn			
Bagby	Louis (AB)			
Ball	Frank L.			
Ball	Orrie H.			
Barber	Leslie C.			
Barker	Jesse W.			
Baum	Harry			
Benham	Charles E.			
Bennet	F. C.			
Bird	John Clifton			
Bixby	Joseph			
Bowers	Harvey E.			
Brown	Charles Phillip			
Burkhardt	Edward A.			
Chapman	Charles			
Clark	Fred H.			
Colt	James D., Jr.			
Cowden/Cowdeen	A. L.			
Cox	Henry Anderson			
Crabtree	R. E.			
Cralk/Craik	Charles W.			
Creel	Richard H.			
Crisler	Marcus P.			
Czarlinsky	Harry			
Daniels	Edmund N.			
Davis	Joseph Edward			
Day	Ernest F.			
Donaldson	Clyde O.			

Surname	Given Names	City	State	Remarks
1900 Continues				
Dowell	G. Shacklett			
Durrett	D. Webster			
East	Theophilus H.			
Eisenbise	Joshua Milton			
Fair	Sheilds W.			
Fitzpatrick	W. T.			
Gillespie	R. Arch			
Haas	Edwin			
Hall	Anson P.			
Hall	H. Eldon			
Hammonds	Oliver O.			
Hansen	Nils P.			
Harkey	William Cathey			
Harris	Carl			
Hays	Henry Everett			
Heller	Harry Lionel			
Hendrix	Benjamin E.			
Hill	William H.			
Hilts	Frederick			Prize (Instruments)
Holt	Thomas T.			
Huff	Boliver			
Huff	W. D.			
Hull	W. Samuel			
Jacobus	Willis L.			
Jennett	Harry Nelson			
Kerr	William James			
Kimberlin	J. W.			
Lacy	Jasper Newton			
Litsinger	George H.			Prize ($100)
Little	Alonzo W.			
Lodge	Athens V.			
Lowe	Robert E.			
Magill	Jay L.			
Martin	Emmanuel N. (AB)			
Marty	Loraine A.			
Matthews	Francis Holmes			
McClanahan	Owen G.			
McClure	Richard Calvin			
McCrea	Edward L.			
Miller	William A.			
Minnick	Andrew G.			
Minor	Preston Hemmingway			
Nylund	Carl A.			
O'Donnell	Alfred			
O'Donnell	Arthur E.			
Olsen	Xenophon			

Surname	Given Names	City	State	Remarks
1900 Continues				
Padgett	James Tressallian			
Porter	Allen L.			
Porter	George B.			
Potter	Harry Evan			
Reece	H. E.			
Rhodes	James J.			
Rice	George Wesley			
Ritter	John Melvin			
Robison/Robinson	William A.			
Rosenburg	Herman			
Rowe	William Guy			
Roy	Frank K.			
Safford	Charles G.			
Sanders	St. Elmo			Prize (Instruments)
Scott	W. J.			
Seckler	Ralph L.			
Seitz	George			
Sheldon	Samuel			
Snell	Lewis C.			
Snider	J. Scott			
Thayer	Herbert S.			
Todd	Thomas B.			
Trowbridge	J. Allen			
Trowbridge	Willis Chester			
Tutt	John Maurice (AB)			
Waful	Mort W.			
Wattles	Junius Hiram, Jr.			
Whitaker	William J.			
Wilkins	Archie Edgar			
Williams	H. Marion			
Williamson	Fulton B.			
Wilson	H. Ross			
Wollgast	George F. R.			
Wood	Orlin Pearl			
Woolis	Asa Lee			
Wormington	Frank L.			
Wyatt	Thomas Eddy			
Wysong	Luther Edwin			
Zeller	Henry Joseph			
1901				
Adcock	J. A. B.			
Beers	E. G.			
Beil	J. W.			
Bickel	J. T.			
Bishoff	M. L.			

Surname	Given Names	City	State	Remarks
1901 Continues				
Bradford	W. C.			
Brinkley	F. O.			
Burney	R. H.			
Campbell	J. A. B.			
Cary	W. E.	Kansas City	MO	Prize (Instruments)
Chapin	C.			
Clemmons	W. M.			
Coffey	G. C.			
Conover	C. C.			
Cooper	J. H.			
Cowen	H. K.			
Creighton	J. W.			
Dodd	C. S.			
Eubank	A. E.			
Feese	J. P.			
Gant	S. S.			
Gaston	C. E.			
Gill	A. F.			
Grady	L. C.			
Grimes	W. P.			
Haas	A. R.			
Hackney	G. V.			
Hardy	I. V.			
Harvy	L. S.			
Hornbeck	H. H.			
Huff	B.			
Hunberger/Hunsberger	H. G.			
Igel	R. L.			
James	Lee			
Jarvis	H. C. or J. B.			
Lewis	L. C.			
Luckenbaugh	A. E.			
Lyle	H. M.			
Martin	E. W.			
McCandless	O. H.			
McCrea/McCray	O. D.			
McCulough	G. A.			
McDonald	J. G.			
Miller	W. W			
Mitchell	G. V.			
Moore	J. O.			
Morley	F. R.			
Moulder	G. A.			
Moulder	J. D.			
Need	Omar U.			
Nylund	G. A.			

Surname	Given Names	City	State	Remarks
1901 Continues				
Patton	W. D.			
Polk	D. H.			
Ray	L. W.			
Richards	N. H.			
Ringel	George			
Russell	E. L.			
Schmid	R. J.			
Scott	M. K.			
Settle	C. T			
Shafer	F. M.			
Sharpe	A.			
Shively	D. M.			
Shumway	J. R.			
Stafford	P./R. B.			
Stevens	W. W.			
Steward	E. A.			
Sutton	R. L.	Rockport	MO	Prize ($100)
Toland	C. J.			
Volp	J. H.			
Warner	J. A.			
Wheatley	C. I.			
Whitaker/Whittaker	J. H.			
Willitts	W. C.	Kansas City	MO	Prize (Books)
1902				
Beals	B. C. (BS)			Prize ($100)
Bishoff	Mark L. (AB)			
Board	Jesse W. (BS)			
Brown	Edgar H. (BS)			
Bungardt	Alfred H. (BS)			
Cross	Walter M. (AB)			
Ewing	Charles H. (AB)			
Gaston	Charles E. (MD)			
Gatley	Perin F.			
Gorman	Henry F. (PhG)			Prize
Helper	Clarence R.			Prize
Kepner	John W. (PhG)			
Lowrey	Claude			
McCullough	William A. (BS)			
McGee	Charles J. (AB)			
Miner	A. Castle			
Morrison	Henry M.			
Nelson	Enos A. (BS)			
Nossaman	Silas W. (BG)			
Nylund	George A.			
Pittam	J. Thomas (PhG)			

Surname	Given Names	City	State	Remarks
1902 Continues				
Porter	E. Marvin (AB)			
Settle	H. F.			
Shafer	Claude L.			
Shultz	J. Walton			
Steward	Edgar A. (PhG)			
Wiliams	Fred			
Wilson	Edward L.			
Yeremian	O. H. (MD)			
1903				
Abell	Charles E.			
Alderman	W. C.			
Alexander	Ralph L.			
Anderson	Eric			
Baker	W. L.			
Bell	Dan H.			Prize ($100)
Beverley	G. W.			
Blades	S. T.			
Blanford	D. I.			
Boone	J. I.			Prize (Instruments)
Cabeen	Robert J.			
Carlson	Ben W.			
Castle	Claude H.			
Cather	Ernest J.			
Chaney	Walter C.			
Christian	R. Ord			
Clagett	Oscar S.			
Cope	J. Q.			
Crowder	William H. (PhG)			
Davis	Elmer T.			
Dowell	H. S.			
Fitzpatrick	Charles M.			
Geraughty	Edward			
Gillespie	R. A.			
Graham	Claude I.			
Hains	John			
Harlin	Robert J.			
Hart	R. Charles			
Hawley	Seth DeZell			
Henderson	James P.			
Henry	John B.			
Hilts	F.			
Hogan	William G.			
Howard	Joseph William			
Johnson	Archie N.			Prize (Book)
Johnston	M. D.			

Surname	Given Names	City	State	Remarks

1903 Continues

Surname	Given Names
Kesner	Gilbert G.
Krimminger	C. E.
Krohn	M. J.
Martin	Roy W.
Mathis	William K.
McKillip	Otho L.
Moser	Edward P.
Moser	Howard M.
O'Brien	Leo A.
Poorman	Bert A.
Ramsay	W. G.
Ratliff	Harry S.
Reeves	E. A.
Rider	Eugene E.
Sams	Louis V.
Sanderson	W. C.
Schwartz	Edward F.
Shore	W. B.
Smith	H. C.
Swann	A. T.
Thomas	C. S.
Tiemann	Theodore G.
Van Scoyoc	W. N.
Wells	S. M.
Whinery	S. C.
Wilson	John P.
Zeller	Charles F.

1904

Surname	Given Names
Adams	Wilson R.
Adcock	Delbert C.
Antle	Harry C.
Armstrong	John B.
Ball	Weldon H.
Beckmann	William
Belove	Benjamin
Belshe	George W.
Benson	William I.
Bills	Richard L.
Burtch	Claude E.
Coonrad	Guy N.
Dieter	J. N.
Dod	Frederick L.
Fleming	George N.
Fortner	Charles H.
Foster	Theodore N.

Surname	Given Names	City	State	Remarks
1904 Continues				
Fowlston	John			
Francke	J. M.			
Garrison	Benjamin E.			
George	William F.			
Graham	J. Dale			
Green	George W.			
Greene	Joseph W.			
Hewett	Sheldon B.			
Hobbs	William W.			
Huber	Albert			
Johnson	Carroll A.			
Johnstone	Paul A.			
Jordaan	John D.			
Kennedy	John T.			
Krohn	Harry N.			
Lake	Noel E.			
Lamb	Joseph A.			
Lawrence	Charles W.			
Lewis	Clemens C.			
Lynn	William J.			
Mackey	John F.			
McMaster	John A.			
Meyer	August A.			
Meyers	Thomas W.			
Moffett	Francis J.			
Morgan	James H.			
Morrison	Lon C.			
Mulvany	Alva B.			
Nave	Henry A.			
Nossaman	Arthur H.			
Owens	Joseph L.			
Owens	Michael J.			
Palmer	Edward M.			
Parker	John Z.			
Pigg	William J.			
Riggs	Lester D.			
Robinson	James M.			
Robinson	Joseph H.			
Robinson	W. J.			
Schoor	William F.			
Schrant	John H.			
Shelton	William A.			
Simon	Ernest G.			
Smith	Dwight C.			
Staver	Benjamin F.			
Stebbins	Nehemiah I.			

Surname	Given Names	City	State	Remarks
1904 Continues				
Taylor	Clifford D.			
Weller	Ralph E.			
Wells	Sanford E.			
Willey	Harry J.			
1905				
Kerr	Cary/Carey C.	Los Angeles	CA	Prize (Instruments)
Lux	Paul	Kansas City	MO	Prize ($100)
Spicer	Charles M.	St. Louis	MO	Prize (Instruments)
Also 55 others				

Newspapers

18 March 1890, Music Hall, 10th Annual Commencement
"Given Diplomas: Commencement Exercises of University Medical College," *Kansas City (Mo.) Daily Journal,* 19 March 1890, page 3, column 4.
"The University Medical College," *Kansas City (Mo.) Star,* 19 March 1890, page 3, column 1.
"Fifteen Young Doctors: Tenth Annual Commencement Exercises of the University Medical College," *Kansas City (Mo.) Times,* 19 March 1890, page 8, column 3.

14 March 1891, Warder Grand Opera House, 11th Annual Commencement
"The Coveted Sheepskin: Bestowed upon Graduates of the University Medical College," *Kansas City (Mo.) Daily Journal,* 15 March 1891, page 8, column 2.
"M. D. after Their Names Now: Diplomas Prsented to Graduates by the University Medical College," *Kansas City (Mo.) Times,* 15 March 1891, page 3, columns 5-6.

22 March 1892, Auditorium Theater, 12th Annual Commencement
"Commencement Exercises: A Large Number Will Be Held during This Month," *Kansas City (Mo.) Daily Journal,* 09 March 1892, page 3, column 6. **(no list of graduates)**
"Thirty-Six Graduates: Commencement Exercises of the University Medical College," *Kansas City (Mo.) Daily Journal,* 23 March 1892, page 8, column 5. **(no list of graduates)**
"Doctors by the Dozen: The Product of the University Medical College Sent Forth into the World," *Kansas City (Mo.) Star,* 23 March 1892, page 3, column 3.
"How're Your Lungs Today? Here Are Doctors by the Dozens to Remedy Any Defects," *Kansas City (Mo.) Times,* 23 March 1892, page 8, column 1.

21 March 1893, Auditorium Theater, 13th Annual Commencement
"They Want Patients: Eighteen Students of the University Medical College Receive Their Diplomas and Participate in a Banquet," *Kansas City (Mo.) Daily Journal,* 22 March 1893, page 3, column 4.
"Twenty Will Graduate: Commencement Exercises of the University Medical College Tuesday Night," *Kansas City (Mo.) Star,* 20 March 1893, page 7, column 5.
"Now Have the Affix, M. D.: The University Medical College Launches Eighteen New Physicians," *Kansas City (Mo.) Star,* 22 March 1893, page 7, column 6.
"May Now Answer Calls: Eighteen Students Graduated by the University Medical College," *Kansas City (Mo.) Times,* 22 March 1893, page 2, columns 2-3.

20 March 1894, Auditorium Theater, 14th Annual Commencement
"New Physicians: The University Medical College Holds Its Annual Commencement Exercises," *Kansas City (Mo.) Daily Journal,* 21 March 1894, page 6, column 2.

"Graduates in Medicine: Commencement Exercises of the University Medical College To-Night," *Kansas City (Mo.) Star,* 20 March 1894, page 6, column 4.
"Nineteen Graduates: Commencement Exercises of the University Medical College," *Kansas City (Mo.) Times,* 21 March 1894, page 8, column 1.

20 March 1895, Auditorium Theater, 15th Annual Commencement
"Thirty-Five Graduates: Annual Commencement of the University Medical College," *Kansas City (Mo.) Daily Journal,* 21 March 1895, page 8, column 2.
"Thirty-Five More Doctors: Graduated Last Night by the University Medical College," *Kansas City (Mo.) Star,* 21 March 1895, page 7, column 3.
"From Students to Doctors: Transition of Members of the University Medical College," *Kansas City (Mo.) Times,* 21 March 1895, page 4, column 7.

19 March 1896, Auditorium Theater, 16th Annual Commencement
"Disciples of Aesculapius: Fifty-One New Doctors Presented with Their Diplomas," *Kansas City (Mo.) Daily Journal,* 20 March 1896, page 4, column 6.
"Fifty-One New Doctors: The University Medical College Graduates the Class of '96," *Kansas City (Mo.) Star,* 20 March 1896, page 12, column 2.
"Fifty-One New Physicians: Sixteenth Annual Commencement of University Medical College," *Kansas City (Mo.) Times,* 20 March 1896, page 5, column 1.

23 March 1897, Auditorium Theater, 17th Annual Commencement
"More Enemies of Disease: Eighty-One University Medical College Students Graduating," *Kansas City (Mo.) Daily Journal,* 24 March 1897, page 7, columns 5-6.
"Eighty-One New Doctors: The Commencement Exercises of the U. M. C. Last Night," *Kansas City (Mo.) Star,* 24 March 1897, page 8, column 2. **(no list of graduates)**
"Eighty-One New Doctors: The Class Graduated by the University Medical College," *Kansas City (Mo.) Times,* 24 March 1897, page 5, columns 3-4. **(no list of graduates)**

23 March 1898, Coates Opera House, 18th Annual Commencement
"Commencement of U. M. C.: Brilliant Event at the Coates House Last Night," *Kansas City (Mo.) Daily Journal,* 24 March 1898, page 3, column 5.
"Doctors Turned Out: The Graduating Exercises of the University Medical College Last Night," *Kansas City (Mo.) Star,* 24 March 1898, page 2, column 5. **(no list of graduates)**
"Medics Are Doctors Now: Class of '98 Is Graduated," *Kansas City (Mo.) Times,* 24 March 1898, page 5, col. 5.

28 March 1899, Coates Opera House, 19th Annual Commencement
"Beginning of the End: Various Colleges Will Turn Out Nearly 100 Graduates," *Kansas City (Mo.) Daily Journal,* 16 March 1899, page 7, column 3.
"Fifty-Five Graduates: Annual Exercises of the University Medical College," *Kansas City (Mo.) Daily Journal,* 29 March 1899, page 7, column 3.
"Fifty-Three New Doctors: The University Medical College's Graduating Exercises Held Last Night," *Kansas City (Mo.) Star,* 29 March 1899, page 9, column 2.
"Enough to Last Some Time: Fifty-Three New Doctors Were Finished Last Night," *Kansas City (Mo.) Times,* 29 March 1899, page 3, column 1.

22 March 1900, Convention Hall, 20th Annual Commencement
"Was a Great Success: College Commencement Held in Convention Hall," *Kansas City (Mo.) Daily Journal,* 23 March 1900, page 5, column 3. **(no list of graduates)**
"Another Use for the Hall: University Medical Students to Be Graduated There," *Kansas City (Mo.) Star,* 16 March 1900, page 3, column 3.
"Medics Fill the Hall: University Students Get a Big Ovation at Close of Their Work," *Kansas City (Mo.) Times,* 23 March 1900, page 5, column 3.

27 March 1901, Auditorium Theater, 21st Annual Commencement

"Finished Work: Thirty-Four Received Diplomas from University Medical," *Kansas City (Mo.) Daily Journal,* 28 March 1901, page 3, column 1.

"The University Medical Commencement," *Kansas City (Mo.) Star,* 27 March 1901, page 2, column 4. **(no list of graduates)**

"Seventy Medical Graduates: Commencement Exercises and Alumni Banquet of the University Medical College," *Kansas City (Mo.) Star,* 28 March 1901, page 12, column 3.

"Small Army of Doctors: Seventy-Two Given Diplomas by University Medical College—Six Nurses Graduate," *Kansas City (Mo.) Times,* 28 March 1901, page 3, column 6. **(no list of graduates)**

26 March 1902, Central High School, 22nd Annual Commencement

"Forty-Eight New Physicians: Graduation Exercises of Two Medical Colleges to Be Held This Week," *Kansas City (Mo.) Daily Journal,* 25 March 1902, page 5, column 1. **(no list of graduates)**

"U. M. C. Graduations: Twenty-Nine Doctors and Six Nurses Stepped Out into Life Last Night," *Kansas City (Mo.) Daily Journal,* 27 March 1902, page 9, column 2.

"New Doctors and Nurses: Graduating Exercises of the University Medical College Last Night," *Kansas City (Mo.) Star,* 27 March 1902, page 9, column 3.

"The U. M. C. Commencement: A Large Class of Doctors and a Class of Six Nurses Graduated," *Kansas City (Mo.) Times,* 27 March 1902, page 4, column 4.

26 March 1903, Auditorium Theater, 23rd Annual Commencement

"To Turn Out Doctors: Two Medical Schools to Hold Graduations This Month," *Kansas City (Mo.) Daily Journal,* 18 March 1903, page 5, column 2.

"To Graduate Sixty-Three: University Medical College Commencement This Afternoon," *Kansas City (Mo.) Daily Journal,* 26 March 1903, page 5, column 2. **(no list of graduates)**

"Diplomas for 63 Doctors: Annual Commencement Exercises of University Medical College," *Kansas City (Mo.) Star,* 27 March 1903, page 5, column 3. **(no list of graduates)**

"Class of 63 New Doctors: University Medical College Graduating Exercises," *Kansas City (Mo.) Times,* 27 March 1903, page 5, column 1.

07 April 1904, Willis Wood Theater, 24th Annual Commencement

"Making New Doctors: University Medical Commencement Largely Attended," *Kansas City (Mo.) Daily Journal,* 08 April 1904, page 12, columns 1-3. **(no list of graduates)**

"Medical College Commencement," *Kansas City (Mo.) Star,* 07 April 1904, page 9, column 1. **(no list of graduates)**

"Many New Doctors: University Medical College Will Graduate Physicians and Nurses Next Week," *Kansas City (Mo.) Times,* 02 April 1904, page 6, column 2.

"Will Graduate 67 Doctors: Commencement Exercises of the University Medical College This Afternoon," *Kansas City (Mo.) Times,* 07 April 1904, page 3, column 3. **(no list of graduates)**

"Medical College to Hold a Commencement: Sixty-Seven Physicians Have Qualified and Will Be Given Their Diplomas," *Kansas City (Mo.) World,* 07 April 1904, page 1, column 5. **(no list of graduates)**

"University Medical College Commencement: Sixty-Seven Physicians Were Given Diplomas during Exercises at the Willis Wood," *Kansas City (Mo.) World,* 08 April 1904, page 1, column 3. **(no list of graduates)**

07 April 1905, Willis Wood Theater, 25th Annual Commencement

"They Begin Work To-Morrow: Fifty-Eight New Doctors Will Get Diplomas at the Willis Wood Theater," *Kansas City (Mo.) Star,* 06 April 1905, page 2, column 1. **(no list of graduates)**

"New Doctors and Nurses: Graduation Exercises of the University Medical College," *Kansas City (Mo.) Times,* 08 April 1905, page 7, column 2. **(no list of graduates)**

"Diplomas to 58 Doctors: University Medical College Graduates' Large Class—Gives Prizes and Banquet at Midland," *Kansas City (Mo.) World,* 08 April 1905, page 8, column 2. **(no list of graduates)**

City Directories

1890 Kansas City, Missouri, directory, page 937:
University of Kansas City (Medical Department), 911 east 10th, J. P. Jackson, Dean, L. A. Berger, Sec.
1891 Kansas City, Missouri, directory, page 863:
University of Kansas City (Medical Department, 911 east 10th, C. W. Adams, Dean, L. A. Berger, Sec.
1892 Kansas City, Missouri, directory, page 740:
University of Kansas City (Medical Department), 911 e 10th, C. W. Adams, Dean, L. A. Berger, Sec.
1893 Kansas City, Missouri, directory, page 745:
University Medical College, 913 e 10th
1894 Kansas City, Missouri, directory, page 754:
University Medical College, 913 e 10th
1895 Kansas City, Missouri, directory, page 663:
University Medical College, 913 e 10th, Dr J M Allen pres; Dr L A Berger sec; Dr C W Adams dean
1896 Kansas City, Missouri, directory, page 704:
University Medical College, 913 e 10th, Dr J M Allen pres; Dr L A Berger sec; Dr E R Lewis treas; Dr J P Jackson dean
1897 Kansas City, Missouri, directory, page 686:
University Medical College, 911 e 10th J M Allen pres; L A Berger sec; S G Gant treas; C F Wainright dean
1898 Kansas City, Missouri, directory, page 967:
University Medical College, 913 e 10th, Dr. C. F. Wainright, Pres.; Dr. S. G. Gant, Dean; Dr. John Punton, Sec.; Dr. S. C. James, Treas.
1899 Kansas City, Missouri, directory, page 1084:
University Medical College, 913 e 10th. Dr. C. F. Wainright, Pres; Dr. S. G. Gant, Dean; Dr. John Punton, Sec.
1900 Kansas City, Missouri, directory, page 1293:
University Medical College, 911 e 10th. Dr. J. E. Logan, Pres; Dr. C. F. Wainright, Dean; Dr. J. M. Jackson, Sec.
1901 Kansas City, Missouri, directory, page 1099:
University Medical College 911-913 e 10th Dr J L Logan pres, Dr S C James dean, Dr J N Jackson sec
1902 Kansas City, Missouri, directory, page 1201:
University Medical College 911-913 e 10th Dr J E Logan pres, Dr S C James dean, Dr J N Jackson sec
1903 Kansas City, Missouri, directory, page 1192:
University Medical College 911-913 e 10th Dr J E Logan pres, Dr S C James v-pres, Dr John Punton sec, Dr F B Tiffany treas, Dr C A Ritter dean
1904 Kansas City, Missouri, directory, page 1226:
University Medical College 911-913 e 10th Dr J E Logan pres Dr John Punton sec Dr F B Tiffany treas Dr S C James dean Dr C A Ritter curator Dr W M Cross clk
1905 Kansas City, Missouri, directory, page 1161:
University Medical College 911-913 e 10th Dr J E Logan pres Dr John Punton sec Dr S C James dean Dr C A Ritter curator

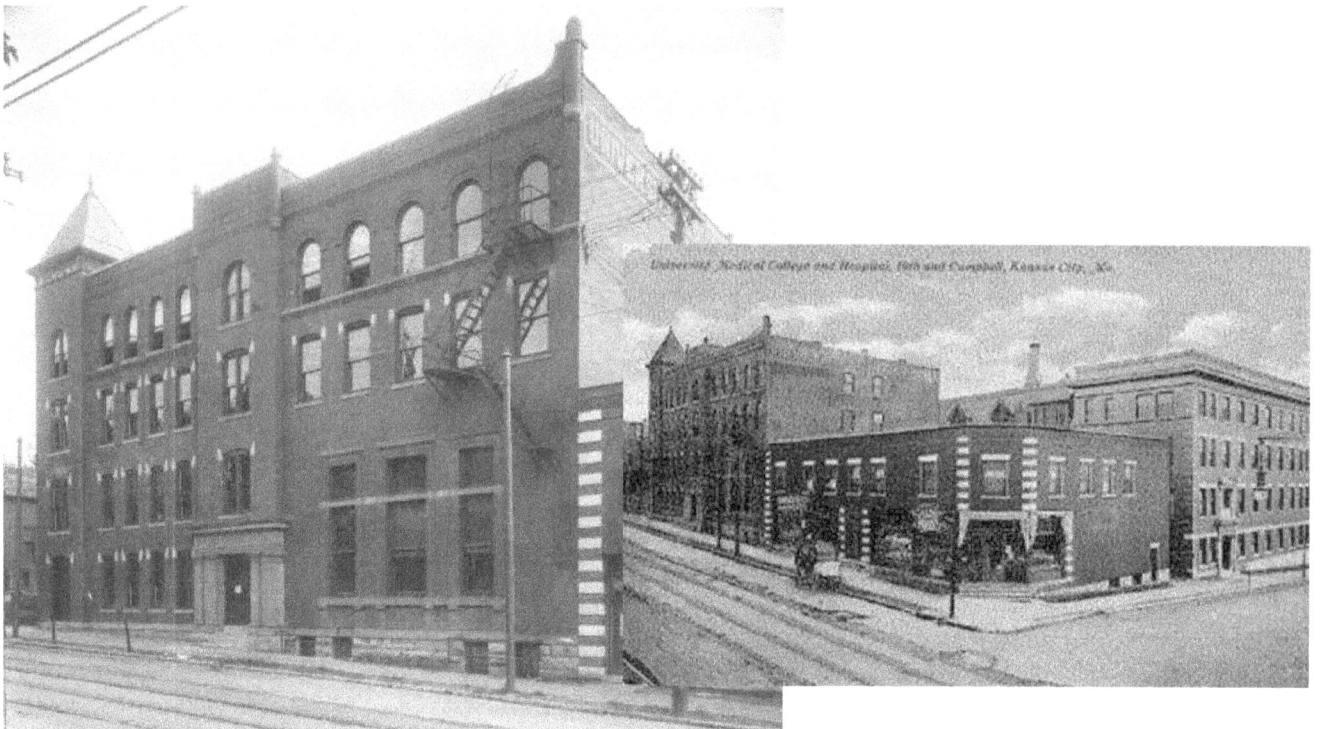

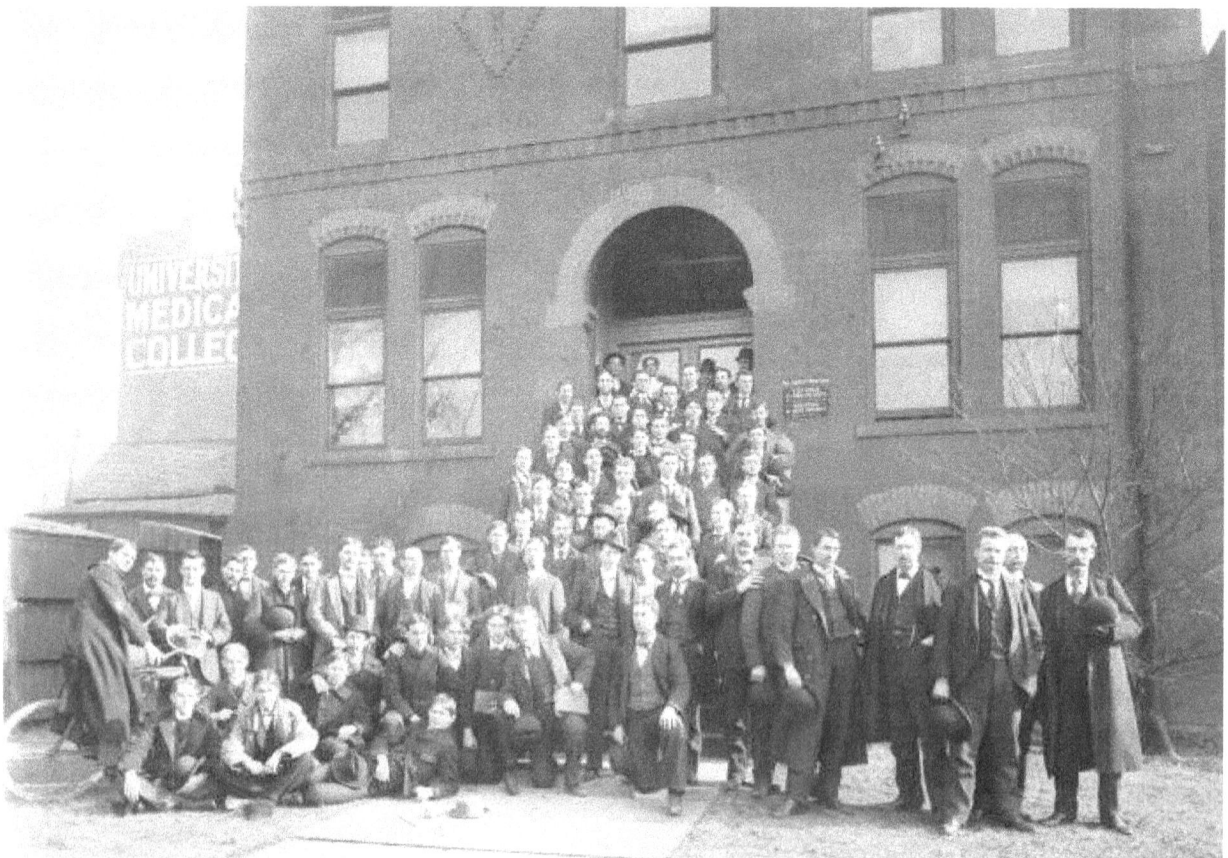

University Medical College and Hospital
Courtesy, Missouri Valley Special Collections,
Kansas City Public Library (barcodes 10002296; 10002296 & 20000050)

Western Dental College
(1890-1919)

Western Dental College was founded in 1890 and its first graduating class was in 1891. This college graduated a few female dentists. In 1919 it merged with Kansas City Dental College (1890-1919), forming Kansas City-Western Dental College (1919-?).

Surname	Given Names	City	State	Remarks
1891				
Brown	S. S.	Chillicothe	MO	
Cromwell	J. H.	Lexington	KY	Valedictorian
Edmiston	B. T.	Prairie Grove	AR	Prize ($50)
Heckler/Heckles/Hickler	Harry B.	Columbus	OH	
Lowry	Harry B.	Senecaville	OH	Prize (Gold Medal)
Lukens	C. W.	Oregon	MO	Prize (Gold Medal)
Nelson	Frank	Olathe	KS	
Ray	J. D.	Kansas City	MO	
Sawyer	C. J.	Topeka	KS	
1892				
Ashley	K. P.			Prize (Gold Medal)
Jones	C. C.			Prize (Gold Medal)
Jones	L. G.			Prize (Gold Medal)
Level	Chris B.			Prize (Gold Medal)
Also 36 Others				
1893				
Bonnell	A. E.	Muskogee	Indian Territory	
Bryan	W. W.	Cassville	MO	
Covert	Clifton C.	Mount Grove	MO	Valedictorian
Cullison	I. L.	Fall City	NE	
Raffington	A./O. D.	Stockton	KS	
Watkins	W. J.	Burlington Junction	MO	
1894				
Ball	R. M.			
Bell	R. M.			
Boyd	Frank O.	Marysville	KS	Prize (Gold Badge)
Bryan	M. E.			
Buckle	E. E.			
Douglas	J. B.			
Downing	E. Burt	Kansas City	MO	Prize (Gold Badge)
Fyler	C. P.			
Gaines	J. R.			
Hawley	E. E.			
Houston	J. D.			
Irwin	Charles S.			

Surname	Given Names	City	State	Remarks
1894 Continues				
Magruder	W. T.			
McMillen	Harry B.			
Moore	J. J.			Valedictorian
Palenski	H. F.			
Pfahler	W. H.	Kansas City	MO	Prize
Rush	H. C.	Howard	KS	Prize (Gold Badge)
Shockey	Lovell			
Sidey	H. F.			
Smith	B. C.			
Stuerwald	C. A.			
Thornton	H. L.			
Tibbits	O. E.			
Wild	Frank			Prize
1895				
Baum	A. (Mrs.)	Kansas City	KS	
Biggs	L. A.			
Bonfils	W. D.			
Bruce	Oscar			
Burgess	R. M.			
Chastain/Christain	J. E.			
Clark	E. W.			
Corel	C. W.			
Daughaday	Alfred	Kansas City	MO	Prize (Gold Medal)
Gamble	B. L.			
Giehl	A. H.			
Hall	W. N.			
Hartley	G. A.			
Hazlett	W. A.			
Henry	E. H.			
Hood	R. W.			
Howell	T. W.			
Lesher	I. D.			
McCarty	E. E.			
McClure	J. F.	Springfield	MO	Prize (Gold Medal)
McGown	T. D.	Golden City	MO	Prize (Gold Medal)
McIntosh	R. D.			
Moore	L. H.			
Ready	R. L.			
Sims	T. A.			
Thomas	C. C.	Parkville	MO	Prize (Gold Medal)
Thorp	B. L.			
Tinker	W. J.			
Woolsey	Irving			
Worthly	F. G.	Mountain Grove	MO	Valedictorian; Prize (Gold Medal)

Surname	Given Names	City	State	Remarks
1896				
Anderson	Robert Chester			
Branstetter	Herman Frederick			
Broadbent	William			
Brown	Edgar Pearson			
Brown	Edwin Sever			
Burris	Clarence Manfred			
Chapin	Willis Victor			
Clark	Christopher Columbus			
Clark	John Logan			
Covey	Russell Elmer			
Dabbs	Edward Abner			
Delaney	Fannie (Miss)	Independence	MO	
Downing	George Whitman			
Edwards	Albert Ulysses			
Ehlers	Martin Frederick			
Flora	William Walter			Prize (Gold Medal)
Green	Theodore			
Hamisfar	Morton David			
Harris	Samuel Wilson			Prize (Gold Medal)
Howard	John W.			
Hunter	Samuel Robert			
Huntling	John Frank			
Jenkins	Evan D.			
Kelly	George Francis			
Kemper	Guy			
Kent	Richard Hiram			
Kirby	William Dillingham			
Lobban	Frank Gilkeson			
Lyell	Thomas Walter			Valedictorian
McBeath	William			
McCrum	Ralph Hammond			
McDonald	Francis Marion			
McMillen	Thomas			
Mirick	Joseph Shelby			
Morrow	Welby Stanley			
Muckley	Omar Preston			
Muckley	Orin Knisley			
Parker	John A.			
Pepper	John Robert			
Purl	Henry Bosworth			Prize (Instruments)
Riley	Harley John			
Smith	Noah Richard			
Smith	Theophilus Paul			
Steinmeyer	John August			
Stuttaford	Herbert	Seattle	WA	Prize (Gold Medal)
Thompson	James Campbell			

Surname	Given Names	City	State	Remarks
1896 Continues				
Watkins	John Elias			
Weakley	Charles Delosso			
Webster	Fred Emory			
Wills	Linsey Leonidus			
1897				
Anderson	Robert C			
Arnold	Thomas Wesley			
Barrett	Otto Lawrence			Prize (Instruments)
Bland	Oscar			
Brown	Edwin James			
Carpenter	Edward Eugene			
Carter	Thomas William			
Cheney	Charles Milton			
Dean	Thomas Summers			
Downing	Mary Eliza (Mrs.)	Kansas City	MO	Prize (Gold Medal)
Ehlers	Gus H.			
Fleming	Thomas Benton			
Hamby	Samuel Marion			
Hamill	Lloyd			
Harlan	J. Amstead			
Harper	John Dott			
Howard	John			
Hunter	Robert			
Keel	Charles W.			
Kretzler	Louis			
Lamkin	Louis Fielding			
Lightner	Harry Llewellyn			Valedictorian
Marshall	Samuel Clinton			
McMillen	F. D.			
Means	John J.			Prize (Instruments)
Metzler	Charles Other			
Miller	Fred W.			
Moran	John Herbert			
Morris	Edgar Allen			
Murphy	Arthur Leroy			
Peak	Orin Harry			
Polk	D. T.			Prize (Book)
Reed	Elmer Elsworth (MD)			
Richardson	James Ira			
Richardson	Will Strouse			
Rouner	David Arguyle			
Sands	Dot Swope (Mrs.)	Mound City	KS	
Sears	Albert Martin			
Shannon	Joseph Reed			
Smith	Lutie Florence	Lexington	MO	

Surname	Given Names	City	State	Remarks
1897 Continues				
Sparks	Edward F. K.			
Swofford	Munroe			
Thompson	Augustus J.			
Van Hart	Harry			
Vandiver	Leslie Asberry			
Vickery	Bert Winfield			
Warner	Marion			
Watters	John Thomas			
Wheeler	George Edward			
Will	Joseph K.			
Williams	Martin Luther			
Wilson	Clarence Milford			
1898				
Beason	May L. (Miss)			Prize (Instruments)
Becker	C. P.			
Brady	Augusta H. (Miss)			
Cannon	Harry M.			
Chamblin	F. G.			
Cleveland	C. L.			
Cleveland	G. C.			
Clifford	T. F.			
Cook	Levi			Prize (Instruments)
Craig	Emmett			
Dameron	E. P.			
Frazier	L. C.			
Gruebbel	G. A.			
Hamilton	C. J.			
Hammons	R. W.			
Harvey	Glea			
Hensley	W. C.			
Hubbell	C. R.			
Huffmann	W. E.			
Hurlbut	S. W.			
Jahr	Frank B.			Prize (Instruments)
Keel	Frank T. W.			Prize (Instruments)
Kelton	T. W.			
Kenney	W. B.			
Korff	R. C.			
Krueger	R. L.			
Litchfield	E. A.			
Locke	S.			
Marshall	Edwin			
McCreery	R. F.			
Middleton	C. W.			
Miller	F. B.			

Surname	Given Names	City	State	Remarks
1898 Continues				
Minter	R. M.			
Moore	J. D.			Valedictorian
Owen	W. G.			
Parsons	R. S.			
Peterson	Ernest			
Rhodes	J. H.			
Richmond	T. H.			
Robison	F. S.			
Rose	G. R.			
Rosler	G. L.			
Schneider	Herman			Prize ($50)
Skinner	Charles			
Souders	F. R.			
Stinson	Harry			
Toelle	Henry			
Wherritt	H. D.			
White	H. P.			
Whittlesey	H. G.			
Wiesner	F. B.			
Williams	A. J.			
Winslow	E. B.			
1899				
Bourn	William M.			
Boyd	Will A.			
Brockman	David R.			Prize
Brockman	Elma J. (Miss)			Prize (Instruments)
Buck	Frank Norton			
Douglass	Elvin T.			
Ehlers	Charles C.			
Ewart	Albert C.			
Gilham	Charles Herbert			
Grammer	John F.			
Hair	Franklin P.			
Harvey	Henry T.			Prize (Instruments)
Henderson	Frank Beckett			
Hereford	Clarence Eugene			
Hill	T. Russell			
Lampe	William C.			
Lovell	J. Amos			
McDonald	Roy W.			
Means	Charles William			
Merrick	Raymond H.			
Nelson	Victor Cary			
Prunty	John V.			
Reed	Julian Bronson			

Surname	Given Names	City	State	Remarks
1899 Continues				
Sloan	Clarence W.			
Smyser	John Ward			
Sterritt	Charles C.			
Taylor	George E.			
VanArsdall	Alexander LaVere			
Weber	August A.			
West	Hugh R.			
Wetmore	Herbert J.			Prize ($50)
Whitmer	Jonas C.			
Yarnell	Edgar P.			
Zeller	Henry Joseph			
1900				
Bennett	Julia K. (Mrs.)			Prize ($50)
Bertenshaw	Herbert			
Blanton	B. Frank			
Boyer	Frank G.			
Bricker	Edgar A.			
Cannon	H. L.			
Cave	Frank G.			
DeJarnett	Hale			
Dimoush	Jacob G.			
Entriken	Harley			
Fields	John P.			
Floyd	W. B.			Prize
Frank	E. C.			
Fuller	Clay S.			
Funk	James W.			
Gaston	E. Audley			
Genung	G. E.			
Gilbreath	Perry F.			
Gillis	James Clarence			
Gossett	Stone			
Halbert	Levi H.			
Harley	Stanley E.			
Hobbs	Eugene E.			
Hutton	H. M.			
Kelly	Bernie E.			
Lamont	Ed C.			
Leverich	Chauncey R.			
Marshall	Warren			
McClanahan	Isaac W.			
McKee	Myron J.			Prize (Instruments)
McMillen	Sam S.			
Mills	Earl			
Montfort	Lena			

Surname	Given Names	City	State	Remarks
1900 Continues				
Moore	Nolan			
Neel	W. Ernest			
Nicol	A. A.			
Raffington	W. T.			
Rhodes	C. F.			
Richcreek	Will			
Robertson	Fred W.			
Russ	W. W.			
Scholle	Gus F.			
Sherry	James T.			
Simpson	Stanley S.			
Smith	Charles A.			
Snyder	W. H.			
Stowers	J. R.			
Taylor	W. E.			
Vansyckle	E. D.			
Vaughn	Marion H./M.			Prize
Voires	Allen			Prize
Werts	C. B.			
White	George R.			Prize
1901				
Allen	F. H.			
Antrim	Ed G.			
Bassett	R. G.			
Bolen	D. M. (Mrs.)			
Bradley	A. M.			
Braniger	E. C.			
Browne	Charles A.			
Bush	W. B.			
Cantrell	L. E.			
Clothier	N. S.			
Cotton	John A.			
Cull	R. O.			
Detert	J. H.			
Duckworth	Will A.			
Eckhardt	H. C.			
Fisher	Theo. D.			
Glass	E. C.			
Grantham	O. P.			
Griffin	O. E.			
Gzell	H. H.			
Hillis	G. W.			
Hinshaw	E. L.			
Holliday	O. S.			
Howard	Russell H.			

Surname	Given Names	City	State	Remarks
1901 Continues				
Hunt	Dessie (Miss)			
Johnson	Frank J.			
Jones	Charles F.			
Lay	J. H.			
Lingar	Charles			
Marks	G. W.			
McCormick	C. J.			
McGee	B. C.			
Mitchell	E. E.			
Nugent	W. H.			
Olsen	H. D.			
Petree	Bert G.			
Rand	H. T.			
Rhodes	C.			
Rimmerman	V. H.			
Rush	E. G.			
Sample	Willard S.			
Shoemaker	W. S.			
Taft	J. E.			
Tanzey	Hugh			
Wallace	G. C.			
Webber	George H.			
Wertzberger	H. J.			
Westacott	George H.			
Wheatley	E. E.			
Zachman	F. X.			
1902				
Allison	J. L.			
Boyer	G. W.			
Burgess	W. H.			
Burrows	George			
Cary	Elwin			
Cater	T. T.			
Chapman	A. D.			
Cheney	W. D./G.			
Coppersmith	A. W.			
Coulter	R. S.			
Davidson	C. W.			
Davis	C./D. O.			
Dicus	Clarence			
East	M. R.			
Ewing	G. S.			
Finley	D. R.			
Fouch	Ora O.			
French	W. A.			

Surname	Given Names	City	State	Remarks
1902 Continues				
Gemmel	W. L.			
Golliday	M. W.			
Grantham	Wes			
Halderman	W. O.			
Hamman	L. M.			
Hanks	Claude B.			
Harris	Loy E.			Prize (Gold Medal)
Hawley	Joel E.			
Hemley	John L.			
Holt	Hart			
Lancaster	H. E.			
Leslie	L. D.			
Love	R. S.			
Marsteller	J. E.			
McBride	Andrew			
McFarland	H. M.			Prize (Gold Medal)
McMillen	Otis			
Miller	S. P.			
Moore	C. L.			
Moore	H. Z.			
Morrison	H. J.			
Musgrave	J. D.			
Newland	A. B.			Prize (Instruments)
Nichols	Gilbert			Prize (Instruments)
Noland	C. A.			
Pendarvis	G. E.			
Phillips	F. A.			
Price	McF.			
Putnam	M. N.			
Raffington	G. N./U.			
Ridgeway	Asa J.			
Riggs	S. B.			
Rinehart	R. J.			
Rudy	L. N.			
Schooley	M. A.			
Scott	C. O.			
Smalley	Glenn S.			
Teague	J. A.			
Tharp	C. D.			
Thayer	James L.			
Webb	George W.			
Weir	F. B.			
West	L. E.			
White	J. F.			
Wolf	G. M.			
Wood	H. I.			

Surname	Given Names	City	State	Remarks
1902 Continues				
Woods	J. P.			
Woods	W. H.			
1903				
Bement	Elbert S.			
Bowden	Walter S.			
Brown	Clifford E.			
Brown	Harold W.			
Bullock	Franklin O.			
Burgin	Frank H.			
Cave	Benjamin W.			
Chapman	Edwin M.			
Collins	Frank B.			
Creighton	Cornelius H.			
Crume	Merna B.			
Ewing	Robert H.			
Frye	Richard A.			
Guffy	Julius			
Gumno	J. H.			
Hedrick	Glen A.			
Hoard	Lewis E.			
Houston	Howard K.			
Hull	John R.			
Hume	Bert			
Ingram	Martin L.			
King	William C.			
Krotzer	Robert W.			
Lamont	Daniel E.			
Lawing	Ernest O.			
Longinotti	James A.			Prize (Gold Medal)
McAllister	Milton G.			
McKeehan	Alfred B.			
Mead	Fred S.			
Miller	Albert R.			
Miner	Fanny Z.			
Munroe	Andrew L.			
Odel	Burd			
O'Grady	John E.			
Rhoads	C. Joe			
Robinson	Rena M.			
Robinson	Vincent M.			
Rogers	Herbert C.			
Rowe	Marvin L.			
Rubidge	William D.			
Schlecht	John H.			Prize (Gold Medal)
Scott	Norton J.			

Surname	Given Names	City	State	Remarks
1903 Continues				
Scouten	Lucien E.			
Smedley	Ernest W.			
Stewart	Benjamin F.			
Stewart	William A.			
Stiffler	Frances G.			
Swanson	August E.			
Taylor	John E.			
Trusty	George C.			
Tucker	Willard E.			
Tuttle	William H.			
Tydings	Edward E.			
West	Ray A.			Prize (Gold Medal)
Wheat	William H.			
Williams	Joseph H.			
Wilson	Frank B.			Prize (Gold Medal)
Wood	Henry C.			
Worthley	Bernie L.			
Youmans	Charles C.			
1904				
Aiken	George			
Aiken	H. L.			
Billings	A. L.			
Blachley	L. D.			
Boyd	J. C.			
Burgin	F. H.			
Caison	A. J.			
Carlock	H. A.			
Culp	A. B.			
Davis	C. M.			
Edwards	Frank			
Emley	F.			
Evans	W. R.			
Forney	John W.			
Fowler	Maurice			
Gish	Wilber			
Guy	Clarence			
Hallowell	Earl			
Hendrickson	I. H.			
Hill	J. D.			
Hillis	H. H.			
Hinshaw	N. S.			
Hood	Perry			
Hrabe	Anton			
Kraus	Charles			
Lind	T. W.			

Surname	Given Names	City	State	Remarks

1904 Continues

Surname	Given Names
Lucas	A. D.
McCormick	W. L.
McGill	Gertrude
McMahan	Charles B.
Millard	H. H.
Mosley	Ray
Musgrave	Arthur
Nichols	J. H.
Oliver	Edward A.
Owings	S. L.
Parsons	C. B.
Payne	J. R.
Schofield	A. N.
Sheaff	E. B.
Sims	J. H.
Smithers	C. R.
Soash	S. D.
Steinmetz	Charles
Swan	Howard
Talbott	A. R.
Talbott	J. T.
Ward	W. C.
Weaver	C. H.
Wilcox	A. G.
Wilson	I. C.
Younger	Gladys

Newspapers

13 March 1891, Music Hall, 1st Annual Commencement
"Western Dental College: Its Annual Commencement Exercises Held Last Night," *Kansas City (Mo.) Daily Journal,* 14 March 1891, page 4, column 5.
"Doctors and Dentists: Graduates of the Homoeopathic and Western Dental Colleges," *Kansas City (Mo.) Star,* 14 March 1891, page 3, column 4.
"Its First Diplomas: Completion of the Western Dental College's Inaugural Year," *Kansas City (Mo.) Times,* 14 March 1891, page 5, column 1.

10 March 1892, Music Hall, 2nd Annual Commencement
"Commencement Exercises: A Large Number Will Be Held during This Month," *Kansas City (Mo.) Daily Journal,* 09 March 1892, page 3, column 6. **(no list of graduates)**
"Graduates in Dentistry: Degrees Conferred upon a Class of Forty at Music Hall Last Night," *Kansas City (Mo.) Daily Journal,* 11 March 1892, page 8, column 4. **(no list of graduates)**
"Masters of the Forceps: Forty Young Dentists Sent Out by the Western Dental College," *Kansas City (Mo.) Star,* 11 March 1892, page 2, column 2. **(no list of graduates)**
"Dentists by the Score: Commencement Exercises of the Kansas City Dental College," *Kansas City (Mo.) Times,* 11 March 1892, page 8, column 5. **(no list of graduates)**

07 March 1893, Grand Avenue Methodist Episcopal Church, 3rd Annual Commencement
"Class of Dentists: Commencement Exercises of the Western Dental College of Kansas City," *Kansas City (Mo.) Daily Journal,* 08 March 1893, page 4, column 4. **(no list of graduates)**
"Six New Dentists: The Graduation of the Class of '93 of the Western Dental College," *Kansas City (Mo.) Star,* 08 March 1893, page 7, column 6.
"Six Were Graduated: Degrees Conferred by the Western Dental College and the Class Banqueted," *Kansas City (Mo.) Times,* 08 March 1893, page 4, column 7.

06 March 1894, Auditorium Theater, 4th Annual Commencement
"Western Dental College: Commencement Exercises Held at the Auditorium and a Banquet Given at the Midland," *Kansas City (Mo.) Daily Journal,* 07 March 1894, page 5, column 3.
"Dental College News: The Annual Commencement Exercises of the Local Colleges," *Kansas City (Mo.) Star,* 03 March 1894, page 6, column 3. **(no list of graduates)**
"Graduates in Dentistry: Sixteen Students of the Western Dental College Get Diplomas," *Kansas City (Mo.) Star,* 07 March 1894, page 6, column 3.
"All Full-Fledged Dentists: Graduating Exercises of the Western Dental College," *Kansas City (Mo.) Times,* 07 March 1894, page 2, column 5.

05 March 1895, Auditorium Theater, 5th Annual Commencement
"Western Dental College: Commencement Exercises Held and Diplomas Bestowed upon Thirty Graduates," *Kansas City (Mo.) Daily Journal,* 06 March 1895, page 8, column 2.
"More Dentists To-Morrow: The Western Dental College Will Graduate a Class at the Auditorium," *Kansas City (Mo.) Star,* 04 March 1895, page 2, column 7. **(no list of graduates)**
"Thirty New Dentists: Annual Commencement of the Western Dental College," *Kansas City (Mo.) Times,* 06 March 1895, page 6, column 6.

02 April 1896, Auditorium Theater, 6th Annual Commencement
"Graduates of Dentistry: The Western College Confers Degrees on Fifty Students," *Kansas City (Mo.) Daily Journal,* 03 April 1896, page 4, column 6.
"Forty-Nine More Dentists: The '96 Class of the Western Dental College to Be Graduated To-Night," *Kansas City (Mo.) Star,* 02 April 1896, page 2, column 1.
"Now Ready for Business: Young Dentists Who Received Diplomas Last Night," *Kansas City (Mo.) Times,* 03 April 1896, page 3, columns 1-2.

03 April 1897, Coates Opera House, 7th Annual Commencement
"More Dentists Graduate: Fifty-Two Young Men and Women Receive Their Diplomas," *Kansas City (Mo.) Daily Journal,* 03 April 1897, page 3, column 5.
"Dentists Graduate: Three Women Included in the Western Dental College's Class," *Kansas City (Mo.) Star,* 03 April 1897, page 10, column 5. **(no list of graduates)**
"Fifty-Two Have a Pull: That Number Graduates from Western Dental College," *Kansas City (Mo.) Times,* 03 April 1897, page 5, column 3.

02 April 1898, Coates Opera House, 8th Annual Commencement
"Fifty-Four New Dentists: Eighth Annual Commencement of the Western Dental College Last Night," *Kansas City (Mo.) Daily Journal,* 03 April 1898, page 7, column 4. **(no list of graduates)**
"All Ready to Pull Teeth Now: Fifty-Two Men and Two Women Graduated by the Western Dental College," *Kansas City (Mo.) Star,* 03 April 1898, page 5, columns 4-5. **(no list of graduates)**
"They Are Dentists Now: Fifty-Three Students Are Graduated from Western Dental College," *Kansas City (Mo.) Times,* 03 April 1898, page 8, column 3.

04 April 1899, Auditorium Theater, 9th Annual Commencement
"More Doctors of Dentistry: Ninth Annual Commencement Exercises of the Western Dental College Yesterday," *Kansas City (Mo.) Daily Journal,* 05 April 1899, page 3, columns 5-6.
"Thirty-Four More Dentists: They Were Graduated from the Western Dental College Yesterday," *Kansas City (Mo.) Star,* 05 April 1899, page 9, column 4.

"Another Lot of Dentists: Western Dental College Commencement Was Held Yesterday," *Kansas City (Mo.) Times,* 05 April 1899, page 2, column 4.

30 April 1900, Academy of Music, 10th Annual Commencement
"Two Commencements: Two Colleges Have Closed Their School Year," *Kansas City (Mo.) Daily Journal,* 01 May 1900, page 9, column 5. **(no list of graduates)**
"Dental Students Graduated: Exercises of the Western Dental College at the Academy of Music," *Kansas City (Mo.) Star,* 01 May 1900, page 12, column 1. **(no list of graduates)**
"Women Won the Prizes: Carry Off the Honors at Western Dental College Commencement," *Kansas City (Mo.) Times,* 01 May 1900, page 6, column 6.

30 April 1901, Standard Theater, 11th Annual Commencement
"Western Dental College Commencement, *Kansas City (Mo.) Star,* 30 April 1901, page 6, column 4. **(no list of graduates)**
"Diplomas for an Even Fifty: Graduating Exercises of the Western Dental College Followed by a Banquet," *Kansas City (Mo.) Star,* 01 May 1901, page 3, column 3.
"Doctors of Dentistry: Fifty Are Graduated from Western Dental College," *Kansas City (Mo.) Times,* 01 May 1901, page 3, column 5. **(no list of graduates)**

20 April 1902, Auditorium of the Central High School, 12th Annual Commencement
"They Will Be Dentists: Sixty-Six Graduates from Western Dental College to Get Sheepskins," *Kansas City (Mo.) Daily Journal,* 30 April 1902, page 8, column 2.
"Will Graduate 66 Dentists: Twelfth Commencement of the Western Dental College Wednesday Night," *Kansas City (Mo.) Star,* 27 April 1902, page 7, column 4. **(no list of graduates)**
"Diplomas for Sixty-Six Dentists," *Kansas City (Mo.) Star,* 01 May 1902, page 5, column 2. **(no list of graduates)**
"A Class of 66 Graduated: The Twelfth Annual Commencement of the Western Dental College," *Kansas City (Mo.) Times,* 01 May 1902, page 2, column 3.

29 April 1903, Century Theater, 13th Annual Commencement
"A Dental Class Graduated: The Thirteenth Commencement Exercises of the Western Dental College," *Kansas City (Mo.) Times,* 30 April 1900, page 5, column 4.

02 May 1904, Auditorium of the Central High School, 14th Annual Commencement
"Degrees for Dental Students," *Kansas City (Mo.) Star,* 01 May 1904, page 16, column 5. **(no list of graduates)**
"Fifty-Two New Dentists: Fourteenth Annual Commencement Exercises of the Western Dental College," *Kansas City (Mo.) Times,* 03 May 1904, page 5, column 2.

[unknown date] 1905, [unknown venue], 15th Annual Commencement.

City Directories

1889 Kansas City, Missouri, directory   —
1890 Kansas City, Missouri, directory   —
1891 Kansas City, Missouri, directory, page 666:
    Western Dental College, 12 w 10th D. J. McMillan pres H. S. Lowry sec E. E. Shattuck treas
1892 Kansas City, Missouri, directory, page 591:
    Western Dental College, 12 w 10th D. J. McMillan [sic] pres; H. S. Lowry sec; E. E. Shattuck treas
1893 Kansas City, Missouri, directory
    Page 601:
    Western Dental College, 12 w 10th D J McMillen pres; J M Gross sec
    Page 658:
    Western Dental College, 12 w 10th

1894 Kansas City, Missouri, directory
    Page 604:
    Western Dental College, 12 w 10th
    Page 662:
    Western Dental College, 12 w 10th
1895 Kansas City, Missouri, directory, page 688:
    Western Dental College, 12 w 10th, W J Brady demonstrator
1896 Kansas City, Missouri, directory, page 730:
    Western Dental College, 12 w 10th, W J Brady demonstrator
1897 Kansas City, Missouri, directory, page 711:
    Western Dental College, 716 Delaware, D J McMillen dean; W J Brady demonstrator
1898 Kansas City, Missouri, directory, page 783:
    Western Dental College, 716 Delaware, D J McMillen dean; W J Brady demonstrator
1899 Kansas City, Missouri, directory   —
1900 Kansas City, Missouri, directory, page 1039:
    Western Dental College 11th sw cor Locust, D J McMillen dean, D L Wallick demonstrator
1901 Kansas City, Missouri, directory, page 1142:
    Western Dental College [illegible] sw cor Locust, D J McMillen dean, D L Wallick demonstrator
1902 Kansas City, Missouri, directory, page 1250:
    Western Dental College 11th sw cor Locust D J McMillen dean, H B McMillen sec
1903 Kansas City, Missouri, directory, page 1239:
    Western Dental College 11th sw cor Locust D J McMillen dean, H B McMillen sec
1904 Kansas City, Missouri, directory, page 1276:
    Western Dental College 419 e 11th D J McMillen dean
1905 Kansas City, Missouri, directory, page 1210:
    Western Dental College 419 e 11th D J McMillen dean

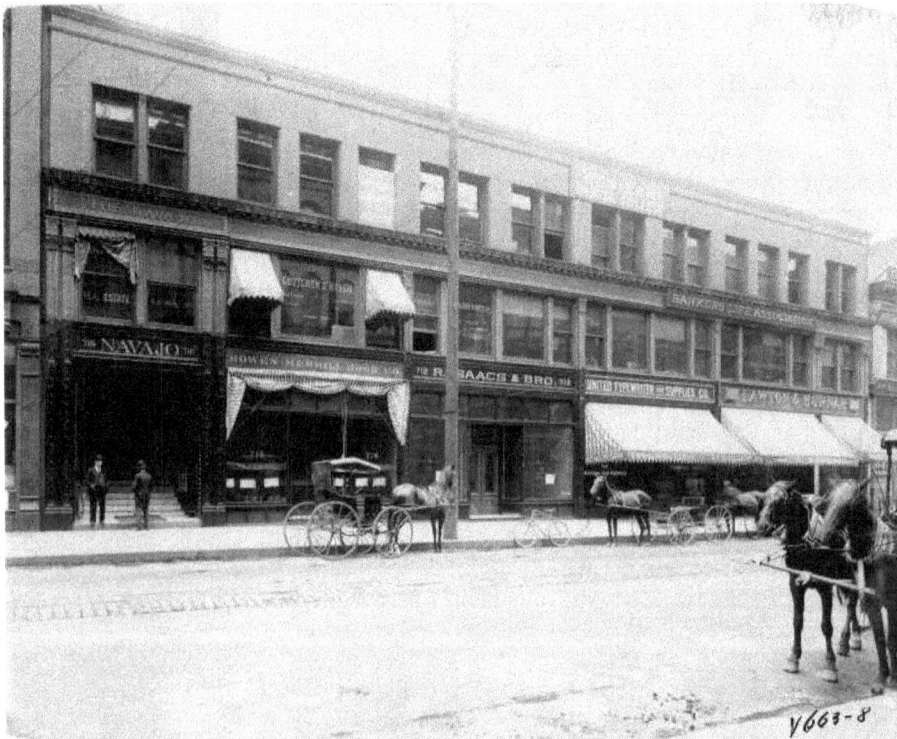

**Western Dental College, courtesy Missouri Valley Special
Collections, Kansas City Public Library (barcode 10001416)**

Woman's Medical College of Kansas City
(ca. 1895-1902)

Woman's Medical College of Kansas City was founded ca. 1895 and its first graduating class was in 1896. It admitted only female students. This school apparently disbanded in 1902, the year of its last known graduating class and of its last appearance in Kansas City, Missouri, directories.

Surname	Given Names	City	State	Remarks
1896				
Metzger/Metzker	Eugenie (Miss)	Topeka	KS	
1897				
Fuchs	Alma (Miss	Mascoutah	IL	Valedictorian
Gantz	Emma O. (Miss)	Saint Louis	MO	
Humeston	Sue B. (Miss)	Saint Louis	MO	
1898				
Agniel	Maude Rosamonde (Miss)	Kansas City	MO	
Branham	Elizabeth (Miss)	Kansas City	MO	
Havens	Jessie Lundas (Miss)	Kansas City	MO	
Lewis	Mamie Pitman (Mrs.)	Kansas City	MO	
Short	Eliza (Mrs.)	Kansas City	MO	
Smith	Catherine Cochran (Mrs.)	Kansas City	MO	
Ziegler	Amelia (Miss)	Portland	OR	Prize (Instruments)
1899				
Board-Bleil	Adeline (Mrs.)			
Farney	Haydee Muzelius (Mrs.)			
Howard	Minnie Frances (Mrs.)			
Murphy	Grace Estella (Dr.)			
Woodrow	Emma J. (Mrs.)			
Woolf	Leanore E. (Miss)			Prizes
1900				
Allen	Dorothy B. (Miss)			
Rages	Nora (Miss)			
1901				
Abbot	Ella (Miss)	Saint Anthony	IA	Prize (Instruments)
Anderson	Mary (Miss)	Omaha	NE	
Morehead	Gracia L. (Miss)	Kansas City	MO	
Murray	Carrie G. (Miss)	Chillicothe	MO	
Peters	Iva H. (Miss)	Kansas City	MO	
Rowland	Mary C. (Miss)	Herndon	KS	
Short	Wilhelmina/Wilhelmine (Miss)	Kansas City	MO	
Tracy	Mettie E. (Miss)	Trenton	MO	
Walker	Callie S. (Miss)	Kansas City	MO	

Surname	Given Names	City	State	Remarks
1902				
Bell	Margaret Jean (Miss)			
Curl	Mattylee (Miss)			
English	Emma Schrieber (Miss)			
Findley	Lottie Romania (Miss)			
Lane	E. Alma (Miss)			
Tinney	Grace Greenwood (Miss)	Kirwin	KS	Prize (Instruments)

Newspapers

16 April 1896, Young Men's Christian Association Auditorium, 1st Annual Commencement
"One Graduate in the Class: First Commencement of the Woman's Medical College," *Kansas City (Mo.) Daily Journal,* 17 April 1896, page 3, column 6.
"Making Woman Doctors: First Graduate of the Woman's Medical College of Kansas City," *Kansas City (Mo.) Times,* 17 April 1896, page 5, column 3.

22 April 1897, Young Men's Christian Association Auditorium, 2nd Annual Commencement
"Three Fair Physicians: Given Diplomas at the Annual Commencement Exercises of Woman's Medical College," *Kansas City (Mo.) Daily Journal,* 23 April 1897, page 1, column 1.
"Women Doctors to Graduate: Miss Gantz, Who Won the German Hospital Examination, in the Class," *Kansas City (Mo.) Star,* 18 April 1897, page 1, column 1.
"Three New Physicians: Graduation Exercises of the Woman's Medical College," *Kansas City (Mo.) Times,* 23 April 1897, page 8, column 2.

03 May 1898, Young Men's Christian Association Auditorium, 3rd Annual Commencement
"Diplomas for Seven Women: Graduating Exercises of the Women's Medical College at the Old Y. M. C. A. Building," *Kansas City (Mo.) Daily Journal,* 04 May 1898, page 9, column 2.
"They Are Women Doctors Now," *Kansas City (Mo.) Star,* 04 Mary 1898, page 3, column 4.
"Women Are Made M.D.'s: Graduating Exercises of the Women's Medical College Are Held," *Kansas City (Mo.) Times,* 04 May 1898, page 6, column 2.

07 April 1899, Academy of Music, Academy of Music, 4th Annual Commencement
"Six Are Now Doctors: Annual Commencement of the Women's Medical College—Banquet Last Night," *Kansas City (Mo.) Daily Journal,* 08 April 1899, page 7, column 4.
"Six Women to Be Doctors: They Will Be Graduated by the Woman's Medical College To-Night," *Kansas City (Mo.) Star,* 07 April 1899, page 3, column 3.
"Six New Women Physicians: Graduating Exercises Last Night at the Women's Medical College," *Kansas City (Mo.) Star,* 08 April 1899, page 3, column 3.
"These Women Will Practice Medicine: Woman's Medical College Holds Its Annual Commencement—Like the Men, They End with a Banquet," *Kansas City (Mo.) Times,* 08 April 1899, page 5, column 5.

28 March 1900, Academy of Music, 5th Annual Commencement
"Doctors Ad Libitum: Many Commencements Arranged for This Week—Programmes Arranged," *Kansas City (Mo.) Daily Journal,* 26 March 1900, Page 10, column 3.
"Women Graduates: Small But Distinguished Class of One of the Youngest Medical College in the City," *Kansas City (Mo.) Daily Journal,* 28 March 1900, page 3, column 3.
"Two Women Graduates: Commencement of the Woman's Medical College—Banquet at the Coates House," *Kansas City (Mo.) Daily Journal,* 29 March 1900, page 3, column 3.
"Women Graduated in Medicine: The Women's Medical College Turns Out a Graduating Class of Two,' *Kansas City (Mo.) Star,* 29 March 1900, page 10, column 1.

"Reed to Women Doctors: County Prosecutor Makes Neat Speech at Woman's Medical College," *Kansas City (Mo.) Times,* 29 March 1900, page 7, column 2.

21 March 1901, Academy of Music, 6th Annual Commencement
"Other Commencements: Woman's Medical College, Homeopathic and Various Other Institutions," *Kansas City (Mo.) Daily Journal,* 21 March 1901, page 10, column 4.
"Nine Women Doctors: Commencement Exercises of Women's [sic] Medical College," *Kansas City (Mo.) Daily Journal,* 22 March 1901, page 3, column 5.
"Nine Women Doctors: They Will Receive Diplomas from the Women's [sic] Medical College Thursday Night," *Kansas City (Mo.) Star,* 20 March 1901, page 5, column 3. **(no list of graduates)**
"Diplomas for Women: Commencement Exercises Last Night of the Women's [sic]] Medical College," *Kansas City (Mo.) Star,* 22 March 1901, page 11, column 3.
"Degrees for Young Women: Sixth Annual Commencement of the Women's [sic] Medical College Held Last Night," *Kansas City (Mo.) Times,* 22 March 1901, page 2, column 4.

24 March 1902, Lyceum Theater, 7th Annual Commencement
"Women Medical Graduates: Commencement Exercises of College Held in Lyceum Hall Last Night," *Kansas City (Mo.) Daily Journal,* 25 March 1902, page 5, column 7.
"Women Doctors to Graduate: Commencement Exercises of the Woman's Medical College To-Morrow Night," *Kansas City (Mo.) Star,* 23 March 1902, page 2, column 1.
"A Class of Six Graduated: The Commencement Exercises of the Woman's Medical College," *Kansas City (Mo.) Times,* 25 March 1902, page 4, column 5.

[unknown date] 1903, [unknown venue], 8th Annual Commencement

[unknown date] 1904, [unknown venue], 9th Annual Commencement

[unknown date] 1905, [unknown venue], 10th Annual Commencement

City Directories

1894 Kansas City, Missouri, directory   —
1895 Kansas City, Missouri, directory   —
1896 Kansas City, Missouri, directory, page 754:
     Woman's Medical College, 1233 Grand av, F B Tiffany dean
1897 Kansas City, Missouri, directory, page 734:
     Woman's Medical College, 1233 Grand av, Dr F B Tiffany dean
1898 Kansas City, Missouri, directory, page 967:
     Woman's Medical College, 1233 Grand av. Dr. R. T. Sloan, Pres.; Dr. F. B. Tiffany, Dean.
1899 Kansas City, Missouri, directory, page 1084:
     Woman's Medical College, 1233 Grand av. E. R. Lewis, Pres; Nannie A. Stephens, V-Pres; Nannie P. Lewis, Dean; Dora G. Wilson, Sec; B. E. Fryer, Treas.
1900 Kansas City, Missouri, directory, page 1075:
     Woman's Medical College 1233 Grand av Dr E R Lewis pres, Dr Nannie P Lewis dean Mrs Emmeline Twiss pres, Mrs Honora Dexter v-pres, MRs E M Taylor sec and treas
1901 Kansas City, Missouri, directory, page 1182:
     Woman's Medical College 1233 Grand av Dr E R Lewis pres, Dr Nannie P Lewis dean
1902 Kansas City, Missouri, directory, page 1294:
     Woman's Medical College 1233 Grand av Dr J D Griffith pres, Dr Nannie P Lewis dean

INDEX
(School Officials in Boldface)

INDEX
(School Officials in Boldface)

INDEX
(School Officials in Boldface)

INDEX
(School Officials in Boldface)

INDEX
(School Officials in Boldface)

INDEX
(School Officials in Boldface)

INDEX
(School Officials in Boldface)

INDEX
(School Officials in Boldface)

Braecklein, Oscar R.: Kansas City Medical College, 1898

Bragelton, J. B.: College of Physicians and Surgeons, 1878

Brainard, B. F.: College of Physicians and Surgeons of the Kansas City [KS] University, 1903

Branaman, Abraham: Kansas City Medical College, 1899

Branham, Elizabeth (Miss): Woman's Medical College of Kansas City, 1898

Braniger, E. C.: Western Dental College, 1901

Branstetter, C. E.: Kansas City College of Pharmacy, 1896

    Herman Frederick: Western Dental College, 1896

    Theron Ives: Kansas City Dental College, 1895

Braun, Philip A.: Kansas City College of Pharmacy, 1897

Breansford/Breasford, G. G.: Kansas City Hospital College of Medicine, 1884

Breck, Louis Merrick: Kansas City Dental College, 1896

Breckenridge, J. C.: University Medical College, 1899

Bredehoft, Julius Curt: Medico-Chirurgical College, 1900

Bredouw, Ludwig Henning: Kansas City Dental College, 1892

Breese, Harry E.: Kansas City Medical College, 1902

Bregoire, Joseph A.: Columbian Medical College, 1901

Bremen, M. Napier: College of Homeopathic Medicine and Surgery of the Kansas City University, 1900

Brennan, Thomas Francis: University Medical College, 1891

Brentlinger, Leland G.: Kansas City Medical College, 1904

Breunert, A.: Kansas City College of Pharmacy (ca. 1886-1898)

Brewer, E. E.: University Medical College, 1892

    J. F.: Medical Department of the University of Kansas City, 1889

    William Philip: Kansas City Medical College, 1892

Brewster, Roger B.: Kansas City Medical College, 1905

Bricker, Edgar A.: Western Dental College, 1900

Brierly, Henry A.: University Medical College, 1895

Briggs, Charles R.: Kansas City Dental College, 1903

    I. Anderson: Eclectic Medical University, 1901

Bright, Henry F.: Columbian Medical College, 1899

Brinkley, F. O.: University Medical College, 1901

    John A.: Kansas City College of Pharmacy, 1891

Broadbent, William: Western Dental College, 1896

Brock, George Griffith: Kansas City Dental College, 1896

Brockman, David R.: Western Dental College, 1899

    Elma J. (Miss): Western Dental College, 1899

Broderick, F. C.: Kansas City College of Pharmacy, 1896

Brooks, Lula Boling: Hahnemann Medical College of the Kansas City University, 1901

    S. H.: Medical Department of the University of Kansas City, 1885

    T.: University Medical College, 1892

Brooks/Brooke, James Frank: Hahnemann Medical College, 1903

Brookshire, William H.: Columbian Medical College, 1901

Brosman, William Henry: Kansas City Dental College, 1895

Brower, Asher A.: Hahnemann Medical College of the Kansas City University, 1901

Brown, Albert L.: Kansas City Medical College, 1898

    Amy (Mrs.): Kansas City Homoeopathic Medical College, 1900

INDEX
(School Officials in Boldface)

INDEX
(School Officials in Boldface)

INDEX
(School Officials in Boldface)

Caldwell, William L.: Kansas City Dental College, 1899

Calhoun, W. S.: Kansas City College of Dental Surgery, 1894

Calmes, James B.: Kansas City College of Dental Surgery, 1894

Calnan, George B.: Kansas City Medical College, 1893

Campbell, Edward O.: Kansas City Dental College, 1903

   George C.: Kansas City Medical College, 1899

   Isaac A.: Kansas City Medical College, 1905

   J. A. B.: University Medical College, 1901

   James Reed: Kansas City Dental College, 1890

   John Malcolm/Malcomb: Kansas City Dental College, 1892

   Samuel T.: Kansas City Medical College, 1898

   W. L.: Kansas City Medical College, 1897

Candler, Fred Day: Medico-Chirurgical College, 1902

Canfield, Herbert H.: Kansas City Medical College, 1893

Cannon, H. L.: Western Dental College, 1900

   Harry M.: Western Dental College, 1898

   Robert: Kansas City College of Pharmacy, 1892

Canoyer, Fenton M.: Kansas City Dental College, 1903

Cantrell, L. E.: Western Dental College, 1901

Cantwell, B. T.: University Medical College, 1896

Carbaugh, Eugene: Kansas City Medical College, 1899

Carey, Clyde: Kansas City College of Pharmacy and Natural Sciences, 1901

Carhart, E. L.: Medical Department of the University of Kansas City, 1886

Carlock, H. A.: Western Dental College, 1904

Carlson, Ben W.: University Medical College, 1903

Carlton, Arthur L.: Kansas City Medical College, 1903

Carnahan, Joseph Lynn: Kansas City Medical College, 1892

Carney, Ira: Kansas City Medical College, 1891

Carpenter, A. L.: University Medical College, 1897

   Edward Eugene: Western Dental College, 1897

   J. D.: Kansas City Hospital College of Medicine, 1885

   James: Kansas City Hospital College of Medicine, 1883

Carrnrae, Lewis, Jr.: Kansas City Medical College, 1904

Carson, L. Russell: Kansas City Medical College, 1905

   Robert T.: Kansas City Medical College, 1899

Carter, Frank Lenoir: Kansas City Dental College, 1892

   John W.: Kansas City Medical College, 1898

   Lew Arthur: Hahnemann Medical College, 1903

   Thomas William: Western Dental College, 1897

   William H.: Kansas City Medical College, 1904

Cartmell, Edwin Ruthbin: Kansas City College of Pharmacy and Natural Sciences, 1901

Cary, Elwin: Western Dental College, 1902

   W. E.: University Medical College, 1901

Case, James H.: Medico-Chirurgical College, 1904

Casey, Fred G.: Kansas City College of Pharmacy and Natural Sciences, 1902

Cassiday, F. F.: Kansas City Hospital College of Medicine (1882-1888)

INDEX
(School Officials in Boldface)

INDEX
(School Officials in Boldface)

Christianson, M.: University Medical College, 1898

Christy, A. C.: College of Physicians and Surgeons, 1875

    Ella C. B.: Kansas City Homoeopathic Medical College, 1897

Church, Miriam Lyon (Mrs.): College of Homeopathic Medicine and Surgery of the Kansas City University, 1900

Clagett, Oscar S.: University Medical College, 1903

Clark, Christopher Columbus: Western Dental College, 1896

    E. W.: Western Dental College, 1895

    Fred H.: University Medical College, 1900

    John Logan: Western Dental College, 1896

    Rolla M.: Kansas City Homoeopathic Medical College, 1893

    Thomas J.: Kansas City Homoeopathic Medical College, 1901

    Zachary J.: Kansas City Medical College, 1900

Clarke, Howard L.: Kansas City Medical College, 1898

    Samuel Columbus: Kansas City Medical College, 1895

    William J.: University Medical College, 1890

Clarkson, J. T.: College of Physicians and Surgeons of the Kansas City [KS] University, 1903

Claypool, Frank J.: Kansas City Dental College, 1891

Clayton, Z. C.: Medical Department of the University of Kansas City, 1882

Cleeton, William F.: Kansas City College of Pharmacy and Natural Sciences, 1904

Clements, Joseph C.: Kansas City Medical College, 1891

Clemmons, W. M.: University Medical College, 1901

Cleveland, C. L.: Western Dental College, 1898

    G. C.: Western Dental College, 1898

    Mary A. (Miss): Kansas City Hospital College of Medicine, 1885

Cleverdon, L. A.: Medico-Chirurgical College, 1901

Clifford, T. F.: Western Dental College, 1898

Cline, Alice B. (Miss): Kansas City Hospital College of Medicine, 1888

    Frank: Kansas City College of Pharmacy, 1897

    Isaac: College of Physicians and Surgeons, 1880

    P. (Miss): Kansas City Homoeopathic Medical College, 1892

    Permelia A. (Miss): Kansas City Hospital College of Medicine, 1888

    William B.: College of Physicians and Surgeons, 1880

Clinton, F. S. (PhG): University Medical College, 1897

    Fred S.: Kansas City College of Pharmacy, 1896

Clopper, D. E.: University Medical College, 1896

Clothier, Mary E.: Kansas City Homoeopathic Medical College, 1898

    N. S.: Western Dental College, 1901

    Samuel H.: Kansas City Homoeopathic Medical College, 1899

Cloud, Marshal Morgan: Kansas City Medical College, 1892

Clutz/Klutz, Ralph R.: Kansas City Medical College, 1900

Coan, Edwin E. N.: Kansas City College of Pharmacy and Natural Sciences, 1902

Coates, Samuel R.: Kansas City Medical College, 1883

Cobb, Fred Lewis: Kansas City Dental College, 1892

Coberly, Lee J.: Kansas City Medical College, 1899

Coburn, Clay E.: College of Homeopathic Medicine and Surgery of the Kansas City University, 1899

Cockrill, Thomas Monroe: Kansas City Dental College, 1898

INDEX
(School Officials in Boldface)

Coffey, A. McD.: University Medical College, 1897

    G. C.: University Medical College, 1901

    George W.: Kansas City Medical College, 1893

    J. L.: College of Physicians and Surgeons, 1878

Coffin, Benjamin Franklin: Medico-Chirurgical College, 1902

    G. O.: Medico-Chirurgical College (1898-1905)

    George Oliver: Kansas City Medical College, 1892

Coggins, John W.: Kansas City Dental College, 1905

Colburn, Jefferson M.: Kansas City Homoeopathic Medical College, 1896

Cole, Hugh Hamilton: Kansas City Medical College, 1905

    T. C.: Kansas City College of Pharmacy, 1896

    T. C.: University Medical College, 1896

Coleman, William Orange: Hahnemann Medical College, 1903

Coley, F.: Kansas City Hospital College of Medicine (1882-1888)

Collins, Davis W.: Kansas City Medical College, 1898

    Frank B.: Western Dental College, 1903

    Helen M.: Kansas City Homoeopathic Medical College, 1897

    R. T.: Kansas City Homoeopathic Medical College, 1900

    Thomas J.: Kansas City Dental College, 1905

Colman, Guy C.: Kansas City Dental College, 1897

Colt, James D., Jr.: University Medical College, 1900

Colvin, Charles H.: Kansas City Medical College, 1900

Combs, Frederick D.: Kansas City Dental College, 1905

Comer, Dent R.: Kansas City College of Pharmacy, 1896

Compton, Fred: Medical Department of the University of Kansas City, 1888

Cone, Norman Homer: Kansas City College of Pharmacy and Natural Sciences, 1901

Connell, Joseph B.: Kansas City Medical College, 1887

    R. W.: College of Physicians and Surgeons, 1871

    W. A. C.: Kansas City Homoeopathic Medical College, 1900

    W. A.: Kansas City Homeopathic Medical College (1888-1902)

Conner, J. A.: College of Physicians and Surgeons of the Kansas City [KS] University, 1903

Connolly, Charles L.: Kansas City Dental College, 1900

Conover, C. C.: University Medical College, 1901

Conrad, Edward Leo: Kansas City Dental College, 1895

    Joseph A.: Kansas City College of Pharmacy and Natural Sciences, 1902

Conry, T. J.: College of Physicians and Surgeons, 1871

Cook, C. F. N.: University Medical College, 1899

    F. L.: University Medical College, 1897

    Laurence C.: Kansas City Medical College, 1905

    Levi: Western Dental College, 1898

    Paul: Columbian Medical College, 1899

    William O.: Kansas City College of Pharmacy, 1895

Cooke, William Fleetwood: Kansas City Medical College, 1895

Cookerly, C. E.: Medical Department of the University of Kansas City, 1882

Cookingham, Darwin A.: Kansas City Homoeopathic Medical College, 1891

Cooley, F[ranklin]: Kansas City Hospital College of Medicine (1882-1888)

INDEX
(School Officials in Boldface)

INDEX
(School Officials in Boldface)

INDEX
(School Officials in Boldface)

INDEX
(School Officials in Boldface)

INDEX
(School Officials in Boldface)

INDEX
(School Officials in Boldface)

INDEX
(School Officials in Boldface)

INDEX
(School Officials in Boldface)

INDEX
(School Officials in Boldface)

INDEX
(School Officials in Boldface)

INDEX
(School Officials in Boldface)

INDEX
(School Officials in Boldface)

INDEX
(School Officials in Boldface)

Hamman, Thomas F.: Kansas City College of Pharmacy and Natural Sciences, 1904

Hammonds, Oliver O.: University Medical College, 1900

Hammons, R. W.: Western Dental College, 1898

Hammontree/ Hammondtree, Daniel Edward: Medico-Chirurgical College, 1903

Hampton, T. J.: University Medical College, 1899

Hance, F. Alroy: Kansas City College of Pharmacy and Natural Sciences, 1904

Hancock, Avery C.: Kansas City Homoeopathic Medical College, 1896

   Mary Belle (Mrs.): Kansas City Homoeopathic Medical College, 1896

Hanks, Claude B.: Western Dental College, 1902

Hanna, Minford Armour: Kansas City Medical College, 1903

   Smith B.: Kansas City Dental College, 1903

Hannah, Jefferson D.: Dental Department of the Kansas City Medical College, 1889

Hansen, Nils P.: University Medical College, 1900

Hanson, Swend A.: Kansas City Dental College, 1905

Harbaugh, Charles Carleton: Kansas City Medical College, 1895

Harden, Charles R.: Kansas City Medical College, 1891

Hardin, Charles B.: Kansas City Medical College, 1881

Harding, Sallie (Miss): Central College of Osteopathy, 1905

Hardy, I. V.: University Medical College, 1901

   James Edward: Kansas City Dental College, 1898

Harford, Daniel Paul: Kansas City Dental College, 1896

Hargis, William Harrison: Kansas City Dental College, 1899

Harkey, William Cathey: University Medical College, 1900

Harkins, Hugh C.: Medical Department of the University of Kansas City, 1884

Harlan, J. Amstead: Western Dental College, 1897

Harley, Stanley E.: Western Dental College, 1900

Harlin, Robert J.: University Medical College, 1903

Harms, J. H.: University Medical College, 1892

Harper, John Dott: Western Dental College, 1897

Harrah, Milo E.: Kansas City College of Pharmacy and Natural Sciences, 1905

Harrelson, Nathan O.: Kansas City Medical College, 1894

Harrington, J. L.: Medical Department of the University of Kansas City, 1889

Harrington, James L.: Kansas City [KS] College of Medicine and Surgery (1896-1898)

   James L.: Medico-Chirurgical College (1898-1905)

Harris, Albert: Kansas City Homoeopathic Medical College, 1902

   Caleb B.: Kansas City College of Pharmacy, 1895

   Carl: University Medical College, 1900

   Edgar Sander: Medico-Chirurgical College, 1899

   H. I.: Kansas City College of Pharmacy, 1897

   Louis A.: Kansas City Medical College, 1900

   Loy E.: Western Dental College, 1902

   M. E.: Kansas City Hospital College of Medicine, 1886

   Samuel Wilson: Western Dental College, 1896

Harrison, Alvin F.: University Medical College, 1895

   E. Lee: University Medical College, 1892

   W. H.: University Medical College, 1897

INDEX
(School Officials in Boldface)

INDEX
(School Officials in Boldface)

INDEX
(School Officials in Boldface)

INDEX
(School Officials in Boldface)

Hornbeck, H. H.: University Medical College, 1901

Horner, Levi: Kansas City Medical College, 1886

Horton, Warner H.: Kansas City Homoeopathic Medical College, 1891

Hough, Harry H.: Kansas City Homoeopathic Medical College, 1893

House, Charles Henry Harry: Kansas City Dental College, 1899

Houston, F. A.: College of Physicians and Surgeons, 1876

    Howard K.: Western Dental College, 1903

    J. D.: Western Dental College, 1894

Howard, Charles E.: Kansas City College of Pharmacy, 1895

    Charles: Medico-Chirurgical College, 1903

    John W.: Western Dental College, 1896

    John: Western Dental College, 1897

    Joseph William: University Medical College, 1903

    Minnie Frances (Mrs.): Woman's Medical College of Kansas City, 1899

    Russell H.: Western Dental College, 1901

Howell, A. D.: Eclectic Medical University, 1903

    David William: Medico-Chirurgical College, 1902

    Edwin P.: Kansas City Homoeopathic Medical College, 1898

    T. W.: Western Dental College, 1895

    Will Waddell: Kansas City College of Pharmacy, 1897

Hrabe, Anton: Western Dental College, 1904

Hubbell, C. R.: Western Dental College, 1898

Huber, Albert: University Medical College, 1904

Huddle, William I.: Kansas City Medical College, 1905

Hudiburg, Walter S.: Kansas City Medical College, 1905

Hudson, Carl H.: Kansas City College of Pharmacy and Natural Sciences, 1904

Hueyette, H. Perrie: Kansas City Medical College, 1899

Huff, B.: University Medical College, 1901

    Boliver: University Medical College, 1900

    W. D.: University Medical College, 1900

Huffaker, Duke Hunter: Kansas City Medical College, 1894

Huffmann, W. E.: Western Dental College, 1898

Hughes, Horace J.: Dental Department of the Kansas City Medical College, 1889

    John Henry: Kansas City Medical College, 1895

    Peter D.: College of Physicians and Surgeons of the Kansas City [KS] University (1894-1905)

    U. S. G.: Columbian Medical College, 1901

Hulett, William H.: College of Physicians and Surgeons, 1880

Hull, John Crawford: Kansas City Medical College, 1887

    John R.: Western Dental College, 1903

    Ralph W.: Kansas City Medical College, 1905

    W. Samuel: University Medical College, 1900

Hultner, A.: University Medical College, 1896

Hults, A. P.: Kansas City Dental College, 1897

    Milton Irwin: Kansas City Dental College, 1899

Hume, Bert: Western Dental College, 1903

Humeston, Sue B. (Miss): Woman's Medical College of Kansas City, 1897

INDEX
(School Officials in Boldface)

INDEX
(School Officials in Boldface)

INDEX
(School Officials in Boldface)

INDEX
(School Officials in Boldface)

INDEX
(School Officials in Boldface)

INDEX
(School Officials in Boldface)

INDEX
(School Officials in Boldface)

INDEX
(School Officials in Boldface)

INDEX
(School Officials in Boldface)

Mackey, John F.: University Medical College, 1904

MacLeod, D. R.: Kansas City Homoeopathic Medical College, 1899

Magill, Isaac H.: Medical Department of the University of Kansas City, 1884

    Jay L.: University Medical College, 1900

Magoon, J. N.: Kansas City Hospital College of Medicine, 1887

Magruder, W. T.: Western Dental College, 1894

Maguire, Edward: Kansas City Medical College, 1900

Mahaffy, G. C.: University Medical College, 1896

Mahoney, James T.: Kansas City Medical College, 1905

Mahr, John Charles: Kansas City Medical College, 1889

Main, G. W.: Kansas City Medical College, 1884

Mainhard, Eugene: College of Physicians and Surgeons, 1879

Major, Clive: Medico-Chirurgical College, 1900

    Sidney Moss: Kansas City Dental College, 1896

Malone, S. L.: Medical Department of the University of Kansas City, 1882

Maloney, Harry W. (PhG): Kansas City Medical College, 1896

    Harvey J.: Kansas City College of Pharmacy, 1891

Mann, Alfred H.: Kansas City Dental College, 1891

Manson, David W.: Kansas City Medical College, 1902

Marak, Rudolph I.: Kansas City College of Pharmacy and Natural Sciences, 1904

March, S. F.: Eclectic Medical University (ca. 1898-1917)

Markham, Robert M.: University Medical College, 1892

Markin, Buyiman F.: Columbian Medical College, 1901

Marks, G. W.: Western Dental College, 1901

    M. F.: Kansas City Medical College, 1888

Marquis, T. B.: University Medical College, 1898

Marsh, Alanson A.: Kansas City College of Pharmacy and Natural Sciences, 1902

    Will Q.: Kansas City Medical College, 1889

Marshall, Edwin: Western Dental College, 1898

    J. E.: Kansas City Medical College, 1888

    Samuel Clinton: Western Dental College, 1897

    Warren: Western Dental College, 1900

Marsteller, J. E.: Western Dental College, 1902

Marsters, C. S.: Kansas City Hospital College of Medicine, 1886

Martin, C. P.: University Medical College, 1892

    Claude Anderson: Kansas City Dental College, 1899

    E. W.: University Medical College, 1901

    Edward L.: Medical Department of the University of Kansas City (1881-1889)

    Emmanuel N. (AB): University Medical College, 1900

    George Samuel: Kansas City Medical College, 1889

    Harry: Kansas City Medical College, 1898

    J. Ross: Kansas City Medical College, 1899

    John F.: Kansas City Homoeopathic Medical College, 1898

    Roy W.: University Medical College, 1903

    W. W.: Eclectic Medical University, 1903

Marty, Loraine A.: University Medical College, 1900

INDEX
(School Officials in Boldface)

INDEX
(School Officials in Boldface)

INDEX
(School Officials in Boldface)

INDEX
(School Officials in Boldface)

INDEX
(School Officials in Boldface)

INDEX
(School Officials in Boldface)

INDEX
(School Officials in Boldface)

INDEX
(School Officials in Boldface)

INDEX
(School Officials in Boldface)

INDEX
(School Officials in Boldface)

INDEX
(School Officials in Boldface)

INDEX
(School Officials in Boldface)

INDEX
(School Officials in Boldface)

INDEX
(School Officials in Boldface)

INDEX
(School Officials in Boldface)

INDEX
(School Officials in Boldface)

Robinson, J. J.: Columbian Medical College (ca. 1898-1901)
   J. L.: Columbian Medical College (ca. 1898-1901)
   James M.: University Medical College, 1904
   John S.: Medical Department of the University of Kansas City, 1884
   Joseph H.: Kansas City Hospital College of Medicine, 1883
   Joseph H.: University Medical College, 1904
   Losson Roisencrans: Kansas City Medical College, 1892
   Oliver Theron: Kansas City Medical College, 1892
   Rena M.: Western Dental College, 1903
   Samuel Sheldon: Hahnemann Medical College, 1903
   Vincent M.: Western Dental College, 1903
   W. H.: College of Physicians and Surgeons, 1872
   W. J.: University Medical College, 1904
Robison, F. S.: Western Dental College, 1898
Robison/Robinson, William A.: University Medical College, 1900
Roe, H. C.: Kansas City College of Pharmacy and Natural Sciences, 1903
   H. D.: Kansas City College of Pharmacy and Natural Sciences, 1903
Rogers, Alfred Hezekiah (AM): Medico-Chirurgical College, 1899
   Elby D.: Kansas City Dental College, 1897
   Herbert C.: Western Dental College, 1903
   S. L.: Medical Department of the University of Kansas City, 1885
Roh, Carl F.: University Medical College, 1892
Roland, Harry E.: Kansas City College of Pharmacy, 1896
   Sarah Jane: Kansas City Homoeopathic Medical College, 1902
Root, Joseph P., Jr.: Dental Department of the Kansas City Medical College, 1883
Rose, G. R.: Western Dental College, 1898
Rosenburg, Herman: University Medical College, 1900
Rosler, G. L.: Western Dental College, 1898
Ross, Harry Reath: Medico-Chirurgical College, 1900
Rothrock, Ellsworth L.: Kansas City Dental College, 1894
Rouner, David Arguyle: Western Dental College, 1897
Rowe, Drury Bridgeman: Kansas City Medical College, 1892
   Marvin L.: Western Dental College, 1903
   William Guy: University Medical College, 1900
Rowell, F. D. (DVS): University Medical College, 1897
   Hiram J.: Kansas City College of Pharmacy and Natural Sciences, 1899
   Hiram Jennings: Medico-Chirurgical College, 1900
Rowland, J. Walter: Kansas City Medical College, 1895
   Mary C. (Miss): Woman's Medical College of Kansas City, 1901
Roy, Frank K.: University Medical College, 1900
Royer, S. L.: Kansas City Homoeopathic Medical College, 1894
Rubidge, William D.: Western Dental College, 1903
Rudbeck, John: Columbian Medical College, 1900
Ruddell, George, Jr.: Kansas City Dental College, 1897
Rudy, L. N.: Western Dental College, 1902
Ruhl, A. M.: Kansas City Homoeopathic Medical College, 1900

INDEX
(School Officials in Boldface)

INDEX
(School Officials in Boldface)

Schlecht, John H.: Western Dental College, 1903

Schmid, R. J.: University Medical College, 1901

Schmitt, G. L.: University Medical College, 1898

Schmitz, Albert F.: Medical Department of the University of Kansas City, 1883

Schneider, Herman: Western Dental College, 1898

    Jacob A.: University Medical College, 1894

Schofield, A. N.: Western Dental College, 1904

Scholl, Grayson B.: Medical Department of the University of Kansas City, 1883

Scholle, Gus F.: Western Dental College, 1900

Schooley, M. A.: Western Dental College, 1902

Schoor, Albert Henry: Hahnemann Medical College, 1903

    Edward/Edwin: Kansas City Homoeopathic Medical College, 1891

    William F.: University Medical College, 1904

Schrant, John H.: University Medical College, 1904

Schumann, Washington Egan: Kansas City Dental College, 1898

Schwartz, Edward F.: University Medical College, 1903

Schweitzer, Julius: Kansas City College of Pharmacy (ca. 1886-1898)

Scott, A. B.: University Medical College, 1894

    Anna J. (Miss): College of Physicians and Surgeons of the Kansas City [KS] University, 1899

    Aretas R.: Kansas City Dental College, 1896

    C. O.: Western Dental College, 1902

    Frank Marion: Kansas City Medical College, 1887

    J. N. (PhG): University Medical College, 1897

    J. S.: University Medical College, 1896

    M. K.: University Medical College, 1901

    Norton J.: Western Dental College, 1903

    S. E.: Kansas City College of Pharmacy, 1892

    W. J.: University Medical College, 1900

Scouten, Lucien E.: Western Dental College, 1903

Searl, O. R.: University Medical College, 1898

Sears, Albert Martin: Western Dental College, 1897

Seaton, George M.: Central College of Osteopathy, 1905

Seckler, Ralph L.: University Medical College, 1900

Secrost, J. F.: Medical Department of the University of Kansas City, 1885

Seeger, E.: Kansas City Homoeopathic Medical College, 1892

Seibel, Richard Moritz: Kansas City Dental College, 1898

Seitz, George: University Medical College, 1900

Seright, J. H.: University Medical College, 1897

Settle, C. T: University Medical College, 1901

    H. F.: University Medical College, 1902

    James Albert: University Medical College, 1893

Sevier, Robert E.: University Medical College, 1890

Seymour, Darwin R.: Eclectic Medical University, 1901

    Sylvia: Kansas City Homoeopathic Medical College, 1901

Seyster, George C./O.: Kansas City Dental College, 1897

Shackelford, Werter Davis: Kansas City Dental College, 1898

INDEX
(School Officials in Boldface)

INDEX
(School Officials in Boldface)

INDEX
(School Officials in Boldface)

INDEX
(School Officials in Boldface)

INDEX
(School Officials in Boldface)

INDEX
(School Officials in Boldface)

INDEX
(School Officials in Boldface)

INDEX
(School Officials in Boldface)

INDEX
(School Officials in Boldface)

INDEX
(School Officials in Boldface)

INDEX
(School Officials in Boldface)

INDEX
(School Officials in Boldface)

INDEX
(School Officials in Boldface)

INDEX
(School Officials in Boldface)

INDEX
(School Officials in Boldface)

INDEX
(School Officials in Boldface)